Abbreviations

ABI: Ankle–brachial index

ACCORD: Action to Control Cardiovascular Risk in Diabetes

ACE: Angiotensin-converting enzyme

ACR: Albumin to creatinine ratio

ADA: American Diabetes Association

AKI: Acute kidney injury

ARB: Angiotensin II receptor blocker

ASCVD: Atherosclerotic cardiovascular disease

BMI: Body mass index

BP: Blood pressure

CHD: Coronary heart disease

CKD: Chronic kidney disease

CVD: Cardiovascular disease

CVOT: Cardiovascular outcome trial

DESMOND: Diabetes Education and Self-Management for Ongoing and Newly Diagnosed

DPOS: Diabetes Prevention Outcome Study

DPP: Diabetes Prevention Programme/Program

DPP-4: Dipeptidyl peptidase-4

DVLA: Driver & Vehicle Licensing Agency

EASD: European Association for the Study of Diabetes

ELF: Enhanced liver fibrosis

EMA: European Medicines Agency

FDA: (US) Food and Drug Administration

FPG: Fasting plasma glucose

FPT: Foot protection team

GAD(A): Glutamic acid decarboxylase (autoantibodies)

GDM: Gestational diabetes mellitus

eGFR: Estimated glomerular filtration rate

GLP-1RA: Glucagon-like peptide-1 receptor agonist

HbA1c: Glycosylated hemoglobin

HFpEF: Heart failure with preserved ejection fraction

HFrEF: Heart failure with reduced ejection fraction

HHF: Hospitalization for heart failure

HHS: Hyperglycemic hyperosmolar state

HIV: Human immunodeficiency virus

IFG: Impaired fasting glycemia

IGT: Impaired glucose tolerance

LADA: Latent autoimmune diabetes in adults

LFT: Liver function test

MACE: Major adverse cardiovascular events

MHRA: Medicines and Healthcare products Regulatory Agency

MI: Myocardial infarction

MODY: Maturity-onset diabetes of the young

NAFLD: Non-alcoholic fatty liver disease

NDA: National Diabetes Audit

NDH: Non-diabetic hyperglycemia

NICE: National Institute for Health and Care Excellence

NNS: Non-nutritive sweeteners

NNT: Number needed to treat

NRT: Nicotine replacement therapy

NSAID: Non-steroidal anti-inflammatory drug

OGTT: Oral glucose tolerance test

PAD: Peripheral arterial disease

RRR: Relative risk reduction

SGLT2: Sodium–glucose cotransporter 2

SIGN: Scottish Intercollegiate Guidelines Network

SMBG: Self-monitoring of blood glucose

SmPC: summary of product characteristics

SRR: Standardized risk ratio

TIA: Transient ischemic attack

TZD: Thiazolidinedione

UKPDS: UK Prospective Diabetes Study

ULN: Upper limit of normal

WHO: World Health Organization

Introduction

The rate of increase in the incidence of type 2 diabetes is concerning, and, although still relatively rare, we are seeing children and young people with the condition. The impact of type 2 diabetes and its complications on an individual and on the health system cannot be underestimated. Now, more than ever, it is vital that all health professionals collaborate closely to identify early, intervene effectively and make every contact count.

In *Fast Facts: Type 2 Diabetes*, we provide a practical overview of this increasingly common health condition for health professionals working in primary care. We focus on identifying and managing those at risk of developing type 2 diabetes, multifactorial interventions to prevent and treat complications, and monitoring recommendations. The book ends with a short chapter on how to manage particular groups, such as older people.

We hope this concise resource will provide readers with the information needed to mitigate the harmful effects of type 2 diabetes. We trust it will help you make a difference.

Type 2 diabetes was once thought to be a 'disease of the West' and a 'disease of affluence', but it is now increasing most markedly in the cities of low- and middle-income countries. Here, people develop the condition earlier, get sicker and die sooner than in wealthier nations. The number of people aged 20–79 years with diabetes around the world is summarized in Figure 1.1.[1]

No country or ethnic group is immune to type 2 diabetes and its constellation of associated complications. Nutrient excess, obesity and a sedentary lifestyle are the principal causes of the increasing prevalence of type 2 diabetes, although factors such as genetics, environmental influences (epigenetics), increasing life expectancy and aging are also important. Obesity-related type 2 diabetes now accounts for a substantial proportion of newly recognized diabetes in the adolescent age group. Over-nutrition has been a leading cause for an increased risk of diabetes, but its effect is different in different populations. For example, South Asians have a genetic predisposition for diabetes. With excessive energy intake and a sedentary lifestyle, these individuals develop central or abdominal obesity. Visceral fat around the liver, pancreas and bowel is metabolically active and contributes to insulin resistance and reduced insulin production from fat in the pancreas.

Non-modifiable risk factors

Age. The chance of developing diabetes increases with age – most people have an increased risk beyond the age of 40 years. The prevalence of type 2 diabetes is highest in older age groups, but there is a rising tide of diabetes in young people. In England, 9% of people aged 45–54 years have diabetes compared with 23.8% of those aged over 75.[2] The age group 65–79 years has the highest diabetes prevalence in both women and men.

In populations of European origin, the vast majority of children and adolescents with diabetes have type 1 diabetes, but in all populations – and particularly in non-European populations – type 2 diabetes is becoming more common in this group.[1]

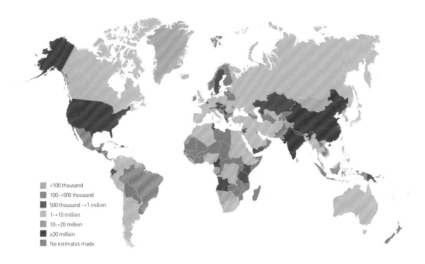

Figure 1.1 Diabetes is a global emergency. The number of people aged 20–79 years with diabetes. Reproduced with permission from the International Diabetes Federation 2019.[1]

Sex. The prevalence of diabetes in women aged 20–79 years is estimated to be 9.0%, which is slightly lower than that in men, at 9.6%.[1] By 2045, it is estimated that 10.8% of women and 11.1% of men will have diabetes.

Overall, there appear to be no differences in the prevalence of non-diabetic hyperglycemia between the sexes.

Ethnic background. Certain ethnic groups have a higher risk of developing type 2 diabetes. In the UK, compared with the general population, individuals of South Asian origin have the highest standardized risk ratio (SRR) for developing type 2 diabetes: around 2.9 among people of Indian ethnicity, below 5.5 in those with a Pakistani ethnic origin and below 5.7 in those with a Bangladeshi origin.[3] The odds for type 2 diabetes is higher for women than for men across all ethnic minority groups.

Comparison of the risk profiles in South Asian and white European individuals in the UKADS (United Kingdom Asian Diabetes Study) shows that people with a South Asian background tend to have disease with earlier onset (57.0 vs 64.8 years), of longer duration before diagnosis

(7.8 vs 6.3 years), with lower body mass index (BMI) (28.6 vs 31.0 kg/m²) and waist circumference (101.7 vs 105.5 cm) thresholds and higher glycosylated hemoglobin (HbA1c) (8.2% vs 7.2%).[3] This is why, in the UK, screening for type 2 diabetes is advised at a younger age and lower BMI for people from black and minority ethnic groups.[4,5]

Genetics/family history of diabetes. Diabetes is a complex condition. There is a strong genetic link to the risk of developing type 2 diabetes. A family history of type 2 diabetes may be considered a risk factor.

Type 2 diabetes is 'polygenic', meaning that it is associated with changes in multiple genes. An increasing number of genetic variants are being identified as potential contributors. There is no single combination of genes that leads to the condition; instead, the expression and combinations of numerous mutations of the problem genes have been associated with a higher diabetes risk. Epigenetic changes that disrupt metabolic homeostasis are now also being recognized as contributing to the pathogenesis of type 2 diabetes.[6]

Genetic variants explain only 10% of the heritability of type 2 diabetes and some individuals with these genetic predispositions do not develop clinical diabetes.

Gestational diabetes mellitus. Some women develop diabetes during pregnancy, and have a higher risk of developing diabetes again later in life; the lifetime risk of developing type 2 diabetes after gestational diabetes mellitus (GDM) can be up to 60%.[7] Breastfeeding reduces this risk. Women have an increased risk of GDM if they have a close family member who has diabetes and/or are overweight or obese.

Polycystic ovary syndrome (PCOS) is a non-modifiable risk factor associated with type 2 diabetes. Of women with PCOS, around two-thirds have insulin resistance and compensatory hyperinsulinemia, which increases the risk of developing type 2 diabetes. This risk can be reduced with weight loss and physical activity.

Modifiable risk factors
Obesity and overweight. Weight gain, BMI, waist circumference and waist to hip ratio are strongly and linearly associated with risk of diabetes; obese individuals have almost ten times the risk of diabetes

compared with non-obese individuals. An increase in abdominal adiposity and a decrease in peripheral muscle mass significantly contribute to the development of diabetes.

Ectopic fat in skeletal muscle, liver or pancreas can distort cellular functions, eventually leading to insulin resistance, reduced insulin secretion and, consequently, type 2 diabetes.

Diet. Any dietary habits that lead to obesity also increase a person's chances of progressing from non-diabetic hyperglycemia (plasma glucose above normal but below the diagnostic threshold for type 2 diabetes) to diabetes. There is no specific food type that causes diabetes, but refined sugars and fat are major sources of excess calories. A diet high in saturated fatty acids and low in dietary fiber, wholegrain cereals and low-glycemic-index carbohydrates increases the risk of type 2 diabetes. A progressive hyperglycemic state is caused by frequent high-carbohydrate consumption – the skeletal muscle and adipose tissue become overloaded with glucose and are consequently less able to take up more glucose. Hyperglycemia thereby contributes to insulin resistance, prediabetes and, eventually, diabetes.

Stress activates the sympathetic autonomic nervous system – 'fight or flight'. Cortisol increases and acts as a counter-regulatory hormone to insulin, elevating blood glucose. Chronic stress leads to chronic hyperglycemia which, in turn, increases insulin resistance and triggers type 2 diabetes in predisposed individuals.

Sedentary lifestyle/physical inactivity is another major risk factor for the development of type 2 diabetes. Physical exercise is a powerful counterforce to insulin resistance. Regular exercise improves glycemic control, reduces the risk of developing cardiovascular complications and improves endothelial function in people with type 2 diabetes (see chapter 2).

Other factors
Depression. Psychosocial factors can exacerbate diabetes risk by promoting low-grade inflammation. Acute and chronic sleep deprivation cause an increase in the concentration of pro-inflammatory mediators in the circulation and can predispose an

individual to diabetes by decreasing insulin sensitivity and glucose tolerance. A meta-analysis of nine trials concluded that adults with depression have a 37% higher risk of developing type 2 diabetes.[8] Depression can also contribute to difficulty with motivation and unhealthy lifestyle choices.

Schizophrenia is associated with increased risk for type 2 diabetes, with a prevalence two- to fivefold higher than in the general population. In addition to common diabetogenic factors, the co-occurrence of schizophrenia and diabetes is also attributed to an excessively sedentary lifestyle, social determinants, adverse effects of antipsychotic drugs and limited access to medical care. Some of the major antipsychotic medicines are also linked to diabetes onset. A genetic predisposition to diabetes among people with schizophrenia is also possible as there are some shared susceptibility genes.

Inflammation. Diabetes is predominantly an inflammatory disorder. The major risk factors for type 2 diabetes (overnutrition, low dietary fiber, sedentary lifestyle, sleep deprivation and depression) have been found to induce low-grade inflammation, which could eventually lead to type 2 diabetes.

Exposure to environmental chemicals. An increase in exposure to 'endocrine-disrupting chemicals' has also been proposed to account for the rapid rise in type 2 diabetes. There is evidence that exposure to, for example, pesticides, plasticizers, antimicrobials and organotins can lead to increased insulin resistance and disrupt β cell function.[9]

Deprivation is strongly associated with higher levels of obesity, physical inactivity, unhealthy diet, smoking and poor blood pressure control. All these factors are inextricably linked to the risk of diabetes and, for those already diagnosed, of developing serious complications.

Morbidity and mortality
Diabetes is among the top ten causes of death globally (see Figure 1.2 for the global picture of the proportion of diabetes-related deaths that happen in those aged less than 60 years). It is a major contributor to cardiovascular disease (CVD) and is the 11th most common cause of

disability worldwide. Undiagnosed or poorly managed diabetes can lead to lower limb amputation, blindness and kidney disease.

Costs of managing type 2 diabetes

Diabetes has a significant impact on health and social services. In England, 10% of the total NHS budget is spent on treating diabetes and its complications, with the highest expenditure on inpatient care.[10] Projected costs are shown in Table 1.1.

Despite the heavy economic burden imposed by type 2 diabetes on public health, prevention and early intensive intervention in newly diagnosed individuals remain inexplicably underfunded. From a public policy perspective, the high costs of diabetes mandate that population programs must be initiated now to combat obesity by encouraging increased physical activity and weight loss for all obese and sedentary people.

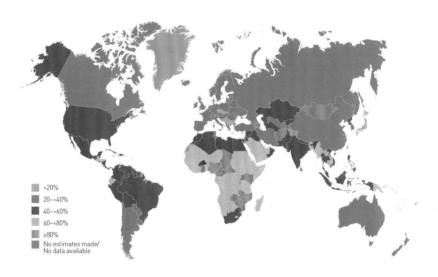

Figure 1.2 The proportion of deaths from diabetes that occur in those younger than 60 years. Around the world, an estimated 4.2 million adults aged 20–79 years died as a result of diabetes and its complications in 2019, equivalent to one death every 8 seconds. Reproduced with permission from the International Diabetes Federation 2019.[1]

TABLE 1.1

Estimated UK costs of type 2 diabetes in 2035/36

Item	Projected costs (£)	Proportion of T2D spending (%)
Screening and testing	17 110 654	0.11
Treatment and management	2 868 489 752	18.98
Prescriptions	1 126 628 120	7.46
Complications	12 224 147 498	80.90
Diabetic medicine outpatients	24 661 589	0.16
Excess inpatient days	3 027 597 751	20.04

T2D, type 2 diabetes.
Source: Hex et al. 2012.[11]

Key points – epidemiology

- Type 2 diabetes affects all ethnicities. In the UK, the risk is highest in those with South Asian ancestry.
- Women who have gestational diabetes mellitus have a high lifetime risk of developing type 2 diabetes; breastfeeding may help reduce this.
- Obesity increases the risk of type 2 diabetes markedly, as does a sedentary lifestyle.
- Type 2 diabetes represents an economic burden that is likely to increase.

References

1. International Diabetes Federation. *IDF Diabetes Atlas*, 9th edn. Brussels: International Diabetes Federation, 2019. www.diabetesatlas.org, last accessed 3 July 2020.

2. Public Health England. Diabetes prevalence model 2016. https://assets.publishing.service.gov.uk/government/uploads/system/uploads/attachment_data/file/612306/Diabetesprevalence modelbriefing.pdf, last accessed 10 September 2019.

3. Hanif W, Sasarla R. Diabetes and cardiovascular risk in UK South Asians: an overview. *Br J Cardiol* 2018;25(Suppl 2):S8–S13.

4. National Institute for Health and Care Excellence. BMI: preventing ill health and premature death in black, Asian and other minority ethnic groups: PH46. London: NICE, 2013.

5. National Institute for Health and Care Excellence. Type 2 diabetes: prevention in people at high risk: PH38. London: NICE, 2012, updated 2017.

6. Dhawan S, Natarajan R. Epigenetics and type 2 diabetes risk. *Curr Diab Rep* 2019;19:47.

7. Noctor E, Dunne FP. Type 2 diabetes after gestational diabetes: The influence of changing diagnostic criteria. *World J Diabetes* 2015; 6:234–44.

8. Knol MJ, Twisk JWR, Beekman ATF et al. Depression as a risk factor for the onset of type 2 diabetes mellitus. A meta-analysis. *Diabetologia* 2006;49:837–45.

9. Song Y, Chou EL, Baecker A et al. Endocrine-disrupting chemicals, risk of type 2 diabetes, and diabetes-related metabolic traits: a systematic review and meta-analysis. *J Diabetes* 2016;8:516–32.

10. Diabetes UK. Cost of diabetes. www.diabetes.co.uk/cost-of-diabetes.html, last accessed 3 July 2020.

11. Hex N, Bartlett C, Wright D et al. Estimating the current and future costs of type 1 and type 2 diabetes in the UK, including direct health costs and indirect societal and productivity costs. *Diabet Med* 2012;29:855–62.

Prevention strategies

In the UK at the time of writing, 3.69 million people have been diagnosed with diabetes (90% of whom have type 2 diabetes); around one million people may remain undiagnosed. Up to one-third of UK adults have impaired glucose regulation (previously called prediabetes and now referred to as non-diabetic hyperglycemia [NDH]). Some of these will have been diagnosed historically with raised fasting plasma glucose (FPG), others by a 75 g oral glucose tolerance test (OGTT); nowadays, diagnosis of NDH is usually from a glycosylated hemoglobin (HbA1c) level of 42–47 mmol/mol (6.0–6.4%). People can go on to develop type 2 diabetes despite having an HbA1c lower than this, so it is important to assess and address lifestyle factors in those with lower values, too.

The National Institute for Health and Care Excellence (NICE) has published guidance on: what can be done at a population level to promote healthy lifestyles; and how to identify adults at high risk and reduce their risk of progression.[1,2] Table 2.1 provides an overview of the key tasks in diabetes prevention.

TABLE 2.1

Key tasks in preventing type 2 diabetes

- Use individual or practice-wide risk assessment tools to identify those at high risk
- Provide brief advice for those at low and intermediate risk and retest in 5 years (e.g. in England via NHS Health Checks)
- Arrange blood testing for those at high risk
- Offer brief interventions to those at high risk but with normal bloods and reassess in 3 years
- Manage those with non-diabetic hyperglycemia – code, arrange/ refer for intensive lifestyle intervention, retest annually
- Consider use of metformin or orlistat with lifestyle interventions
- Add those with type 2 diabetes to the diabetes register

Source: NICE 2017.[2]

Identification of those at high risk

NICE recommends a two-step process for identifying those with NDH or type 2 diabetes.

- Identify those likely to be at high risk of developing type 2 diabetes using individual or practice-wide risk assessment tools (Table 2.2).
- Undertake blood tests to confirm type 2 diabetes or NDH in those identified as being at highest risk using the tools.

In England, this screening process is built into the NHS Health Checks for those aged 40–74 years. A validated computer risk assessment tool can also be used (e.g. Leicester Practice Diabetes Risk Score or Cambridge Diabetes Risk Score) to search the electronic records' database and identify those with increased risk who require blood testing. For individuals from high-risk black and minority ethnic backgrounds, testing should begin from age 25 if the body mass index (BMI) is 23 or higher.[2] Risk tools are poor at predicting risk in these groups, so a blood test should be offered.

People can quantify their own risk using the Diabetes UK 'Know your Risk' calculator (riskscore.diabetes.org.uk/start), or a QDiabetes risk score can be completed in a consultation.

Blood tests. Historically, prediabetes was diagnosed using an FPG value or a 75 g OGTT; HbA1c is now used unless it is likely to give an inaccurate result for an individual (Table 2.3). All individuals identified as having NDH by these tests (Table 2.4) are at increased risk of developing type 2 diabetes.

TABLE 2.2

Groups at increased risk

- Age >40 years
- Overweight, obese or centrally obese (using ethnically appropriate body mass index and waist circumference)
- Parent or sibling with diabetes
- Hypertension, hyperlipidemia or coronary heart disease
- Previous gestational diabetes, baby with birth weight >4 kg or polycystic ovary syndrome
- South Asian, Chinese, African-Caribbean, black African and other high-risk black and minority ethnic groups

Source: NICE 2017.[2]

TABLE 2.3

Individuals for whom HbA1c is not an appropriate initial test*

- All children and young people
- Individuals whose symptoms of diabetes have occurred for <2 months
- Individuals at high risk who are acutely ill (e.g. needing hospital admission)
- Individuals taking medication that may cause a rapid increase in glucose (e.g. steroids, antipsychotics)
- Individuals with acute pancreatic damage or who have had pancreatic surgery
- Pregnant women
- Individuals with genetic, hematologic or illness-related factors that influence HbA1c and its measurement[†]

*Fasting plasma glucose is a better test. [†]See Annex 1 of WHO 2011.[3]
HbA1c, glycosylated hemoglobin.
Source: Diabetes UK.[4]

The three diagnostic methods identify different people, but there is overlap (Figure 2.1). The closer the test result is to the type 2 diabetes threshold (see Table 2.4), the greater the risk of progression to diabetes. Historically, up to 50% of those with impaired glucose tolerance (IGT) progressed to type 2 diabetes within 10 years. However, progression in those diagnosed with impaired glucose regulation (HbA1c) is less clear; in some, blood glucose regresses to a normal (no diabetes) level.

Women with previous gestational diabetes mellitus. Around 60% of these women will develop type 2 diabetes depending on the diagnostic criteria used for gestational diabetes mellitus (GDM) – risk is highest in the first 5–10 years after pregnancy and then plateaus.[5,6] Measure FPG 6–13 weeks after delivery:
- if normal (<6 mmol/L), continue lifestyle advice and measure HbA1c annually to identify ongoing risk of NDH and type 2 diabetes
- if 6.0–6.9 mmol/L, manage as NDH
- if 7.0 mmol/L or higher, type 2 diabetes is likely.[7]

If tested after 13 weeks, fasting glucose or HbA1c can be used (if HbA1c is in the range 39–47 mmol/mol, manage as for NDH).

TABLE 2.4

Diagnostic thresholds for types of NDH and type 2 diabetes (UK)

HbA1c, mmol/ mol (%)	FPG, mmol/L	OGTT 2 h glucose post load, mmol/L	Identifies
42–47 (6–6.4)			Impaired glucose regulation/NDH
	5.5–6.9		Impaired fasting glycemia
		7.8–11.0	Impaired glucose tolerance
≥48 (6.5)	≥7.0	≥11.1	Type 2 diabetes*

*In an individual with symptoms (e.g. polyuria, polydipsia), only one test is required to diagnose type 2 diabetes; in the absence of symptoms, two tests are needed.
FPG, fasting plasma glucose; h, hours; HbA1c, glycosylated hemoglobin; NDH, non-diabetic hyperglycemia; OGTT, oral glucose tolerance test.

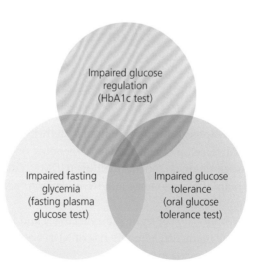

Figure 2.1 Overlap between different types of non-diabetic hyperglycemia.

Risk scores divide people into low-, intermediate- and high-risk groups (Figure 2.2). Onset of NDH and type 2 diabetes occurs at lower BMIs and younger ages in Asian, black and other minority ethnic groups. Consequently, people in these groups who are aged 25 or older with BMI at 23 kg/m² or over should be offered blood testing, as risk scores are not strongly predictive. As these individuals are two to four times more likely to develop type 2 diabetes, it is beneficial to identify them and offer behavior-change programs early.

Behavior change

Where lifestyle advice is recommended (Figure 2.2), discuss the individual's risk of developing diabetes and the benefits of a healthy lifestyle; offer help to modify individual risk factors.

Brief intervention involves signposting to tailored support that uses evidence-based behavior-change techniques – particularly for weight loss (e.g. walking programs, exercise on prescription and commercial weight loss programs).

Intensive lifestyle-change program. The individual should be referred to a quality-assured intensive lifestyle-change program, such as the Healthier You: NHS Diabetes Prevention Programme (NHS DPP) for those with NDH. This should:[2]
- include ongoing tailored advice, support and encouragement to help people achieve
  - at least 150 minutes of moderate-intensity physical activity per week
  - gradual weight loss and maintenance of healthy BMI
  - increased consumption of wholegrains, vegetables and high-fiber foods
  - reduced intake of total fat and saturated fat
- use established behavior-change techniques including
  - information provision
  - an exploration of reasons for wanting to change and confidence to change
  - goal setting
  - action planning
  - coping
  - relapse planning.

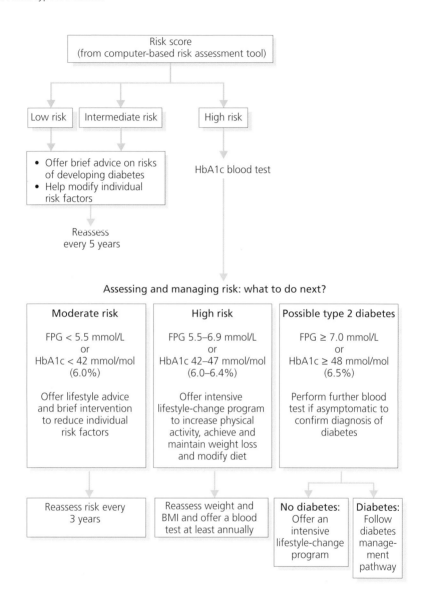

Figure 2.2 Assessing and managing risk. It is important to remember that 'low risk' is not equivalent to 'no risk' – a person may be predisposed but has not yet reached the HbA1c threshold for higher risk. BMI, body mass index; FPG, fasting plasma glucose; HbA1c, glycosylated hemoglobin. Adapted from NICE 2012.[2]

Metformin and orlistat

Both metformin and orlistat facilitate weight loss and reduce the risk of NDH progression to type 2 diabetes.

Metformin reduced the development of diabetes over 15 years in the US DPP (Diabetes Prevention Program) and DPOS (Diabetes Prevention Outcome Study), with most benefit in those with higher glucose or HbA1c at baseline and in women with a history of GDM.[8] NICE allows metformin use to support lifestyle changes in those whose HbA1c continues to deteriorate despite intensive lifestyle intervention or where they are unable to participate in a lifestyle program.[2] Metformin should be considered particularly in those with a BMI above 35 kg/m^2. Therapy should be individualized and the benefits and risks of lifestyle versus drug fully discussed. Check estimated glomerular filtration rate (eGFR) prior to metformin initiation and twice yearly thereafter.

Start the individual at 500 mg daily and increase, as tolerated, to 1 g twice daily. If eGFR drops to less than 45 mL/min/1.73 m^2, reduce the dose by half. If eGFR drops to below 30 mL/min/1.73 m^2, stop metformin.

If the individual is intolerant, consider a modified-release formulation. Only modified-release metformin is licensed for diabetes prevention, so standard metformin is used off license and the patient must be counselled accordingly. Prescribe for 6–12 months initially and check HbA1c every 3–6 months. Metformin can facilitate weight loss and may reduce cardiovascular disease risk as well as HbA1c.

Orlistat can be considered alongside lifestyle interventions in those with NDH and a BMI of 28 kg/m^2 or above as part of an overall plan to help manage obesity.[2] Discuss the potential benefits and side effects of orlistat, and advise the individual to follow a low-fat diet (< 30% energy as fat, divided between three meals per day). Agree a weight loss goal and offer support and resources to aid weight loss. NICE recommends reviewing progress at 12 weeks and considering discontinuing if the individual has achieved weight loss of less than 5%. However, in practice, orlistat, if tolerated, would probably be continued. Weight loss may be more difficult in those with NDH and type 2 diabetes so a longer interval may be required to see whether weight loss has occurred.

Many people will not tolerate orlistat because of the fatty stools and leakage that occur with malabsorption. Encouraging intermittent use (e.g. when not working) can be helpful. Fat-soluble vitamins should be supplemented if long-term use is achievable. Have a further discussion regarding benefits and risks at 12 months.

Practice diabetes prevention plans

Within practices, it is important to agree a strategy for diagnosing and managing NDH to complement the NHS Health Checks or if there is no access to the checks. Ensure those diagnosed with NDH (and all those with HbA1c 42–47 mmol/mol from opportunistic blood testing) are coded and that annual testing occurs. Ensure those historically diagnosed using FPG or OGTT are added to the register for annual testing, as well as women with previous GDM.

Those who have not attended their NHS Health Check should have an alert added so they can be assessed opportunistically when they consult for other reasons – blood tests should be organized if they have a high risk score. Ensure everyone who reviews blood results is aware of NDH and the need to code accurately and that these people require lifestyle advice and follow-up.

Agree how people with NDH will be managed if you do not have access to the NHS DPP. All individuals will need lifestyle advice (one to one or in a group) as well as baseline measurements. Consider including waist circumference for those with a BMI below 35 kg/m², as this helps to further quantify risk, is easy to measure and monitor at home and changes faster than weight or BMI with lifestyle change, meaning it is also a motivational tool. Measure at the mid-point between rib margin and iliac crest (this may be the level of umbilicus).

Macrovascular complications can develop even in those with NDH; at diagnosis of type 2 diabetes, around half of people already have microvascular or macrovascular complications, so monitor cardiovascular risk factors and manage as appropriate.

Stratify risk and ensure that those at highest risk (HbA1c 44–47 mmol/mol) are prioritized for management if you or your local program are not able to manage the whole population immediately.[2] Agree when metformin or orlistat will be offered and how monitoring will take place for those taking these drugs. Ensure a robust protocol for annual repeat blood testing of those at risk and prompt management of those who develop type 2 diabetes.

Many vulnerable adults, including those with psychosis and severe mental health problems, are at high risk of NDH and type 2 diabetes.

Many resources are available to guide management of NDH. Explore what is available locally and what is being used in the NHS DPP if you have access (https://preventing-diabetes.co.uk/).

Evidence to support prevention strategies

The US DPP[9] and the Finnish Diabetes Prevention Study[10] demonstrated a 58% reduction in type 2 diabetes in high-risk individuals receiving an intensive lifestyle intervention and a 31% reduction with metformin. The benefit could be maintained long term.[11-13]

Participants in the US DPP with IGT or impaired fasting glycemia (IFG) were randomized to receive:

- standard diet and exercise advice (placebo)
- metformin 850 mg twice daily with standard diet and exercise advice
- intensive lifestyle advice, with the aim of losing 7% body weight, restricting energy intake to 1200–1800 kcal/day, restricting dietary fat to less than 25% of daily energy intake and undertaking more than 150 minutes of physical activity per week.[9]

After a mean of 2.8 years, compared with the placebo group, those following the intensive lifestyle advice had a 58% reduction in type 2 diabetes while those in the metformin group had a 31% reduction – the crude incidence of diabetes in the three groups is shown in Figure 2.3. Similar results were achieved in the Finnish Diabetes Prevention Study.

In the DPOS follow-up of the US DPP, the control and intervention groups were followed for a further 15 years and all received ongoing lifestyle advice. Despite both groups receiving the same guidance, a 34% reduction in development of type 2 diabetes persisted at 10 years, with a 27% reduction at 15 years, in those originally in the intensive lifestyle group, compared with those in the control group.

Using a risk-prediction model to estimate the benefits of metformin and intensive lifestyle changes on risk reduction in different groups demonstrates benefit for lifestyle in all the risk quartiles, though the greatest impact is in those at greatest risk (number needed to treat [NNT] over 3 years: 3.5 in highest-risk quartile vs 20.4 in the lowest quartile).[13] Metformin reduced type 2 diabetes most significantly in those in the top quartile of risk, producing a 21.4% absolute risk reduction (NNT 4.6 over 3 years), with a much smaller benefit across

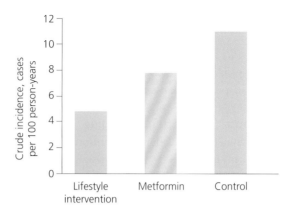

Figure 2.3 Crude incidence of type 2 diabetes in the US Diabetes Prevention Program. Data are from Diabetes Prevention Program Research Group 2002.[9]

the lower risk groups. In the updated NICE guidance, those at greatest risk are to be prioritized; intensive lifestyle intervention is recommended for everyone and metformin is particularly recommended for use in those with a BMI above $35 \, kg/m^2$, deteriorating HbA1c or previous gestational diabetes.[2] The risk prediction model identified FPG as the strongest predictor of type 2 diabetes development and that HbA1c and self-reported hyperglycemia were also independent risk factors, as were waist circumference, height and waist to hip ratio.[14]

HbA1c is now used for defining NDH and for diagnosing type 2 diabetes, so it is important to ascertain if this, rather than an OGTT, is an appropriate way to identify those at high risk of developing type 2 diabetes. In addition to the OGTT values presented in the original paper, the US DPP and DPOS measured HbA1c at baseline and for diagnosis of type 2 diabetes – these data were analyzed in a separate study.[15] Baseline HbA1c predicted type 2 diabetes risk, validating use of this measure for identifying NDH. If an HbA1c threshold of 48 mmol/mol was used for diabetes diagnosis, metformin and intensive lifestyle intervention resulted in similar reductions in type 2 diabetes, 44% and 49%, respectively, during the US DPP and 38% and 29% during the DPOS. This contrasts with the use of glucose measurements for type 2 diabetes diagnosis, where lifestyle intervention was almost twice as effective (29% metformin and 51% intensive lifestyle intervention, respectively) during the US DPP.

Long-term effects. The proposed long-term impact of the ongoing Healthier You, the NHS DPP, has been challenged.[16] The publication of the 23-year follow-up of the Da Qing diabetes prevention study demonstrating reductions in cardiovascular and all-cause mortality as well as type 2 diabetes reduction following a 6-year lifestyle program, however, provides hope that long-term impact may be possible.[17,18] Weight loss correlates with and is an important contributor to prevention of NDH progression, so perhaps this should be the pragmatic goal going forward.

Key points – prevention strategies

- In England, NHS Health Checks screen for cardiometabolic risk in those without cardiovascular disease aged 40–74 every 5 years and will identify those with non-diabetic hyperglycemia (NDH) (and new type 2 diabetes) and refer them to the Healthier You: NHS Diabetes Prevention Programme. Elsewhere, the National Institute for Health and Care Excellence (NICE) makes recommendations on how to identify and manage NDH.
- NICE recommends a two-step process – using practice-based or individual risk scores to identify who is at risk then carrying out blood tests only in those at high risk to identify NDH and type 2 diabetes.
- Risk scores are poor at identifying high-risk individuals in some ethnic groups; a blood test is recommended for these individuals.
- A glycosylated hemoglobin (HbA1c) of 42–47 mmol/mol identifies those with NDH and is the recommended test in the UK. These people are at high risk of developing type 2 diabetes.
- In those with impaired fasting glycemia/impaired glucose tolerance in the US Diabetes Prevention Program and Finnish Diabetes Prevention Study, intensive lifestyle intervention reduced the risk of developing type 2 diabetes by 58% and metformin reduced the risk by 31%.
- Lifestyle and metformin impact differently on high-risk groups depending on whether they are identified by HbA1c or oral glucose tolerance test.
- Ensure people with NDH and previous gestational diabetes are coded and have an annual HbA1c test to exclude type 2 diabetes.

Based on these findings, NICE guidance recommends the implementation of evidence-based validated intensive lifestyle programs such as the NHS DPP as the mainstay of NDH management.[2] Intensive lifestyle programs are now offered to high-risk individuals across most of England. Other parts of the UK are implementing similar lifestyle programs more gradually.

In the real world, it is unlikely that programs are able to provide such intensive intervention and follow-up as in the formal prevention studies. Where there is no access to the NHS DPP, practices should signpost to a variety of services such as exercise on prescription, level 2 and 3 weight management services and dietitian programs (Table 2.5).

TABLE 2.5

What works for prevention in the real world?

- Women do better than men, but there is no significant age difference
- Individuals with higher BMI and higher HbA1c may gain more benefit from intensive lifestyle management
- Programs closely mimicking NICE recommendations are more effective
- Groups of 10–15 are better than smaller groups
- Programs including diet and physical activity result in additional weight loss versus programs with physical activity alone
- Supervised physical activity sessions are better than recommendations only
- A 9–18-month program of sessions is better than a shorter program
- 1–2-hour sessions are better than shorter sessions
- Having 13+ sessions is better than having <8 sessions
- At least 16 hours of contact is optimal, with each additional hour increasing benefit
- Commercial weight management programs may be better than those offered by primary care

BMI, body mass index; HbA1c, glycosylated hemoglobin; NICE, National Institute for Health and Care Excellence. Source: Public Health England 2015.[19]

References

1. National Institute for Health and Care Excellence. Type 2 diabetes prevention: population and community-level interventions: PH35. London: NICE, 2011.

2. National Institute for Health and Care Excellence. Type 2 diabetes: prevention in people at high risk: PH38. London: NICE, 2012, updated 2017.

3. World Health Organization. Use of glycated haemoglobin (HbA1c) in the diagnosis of diabetes mellitus. Geneva: WHO, 2011.

4. Diabetes UK. Diagnostic criteria for diabetes. www.diabetes.org.uk/professionals/position-statements-reports/diagnosis-ongoing-management-monitoring/new_diagnostic_criteria_for_diabetes, last accessed 3 July 2020.

5. Kim C, Newton K, Knoff R. Gestational diabetes and the incidence of type 2 diabetes. *Diabetes Care* 2002;25:1862–8.

6. Noctor E, Dunne F. Type 2 diabetes after gestational diabetes: The influence of changing diagnostic criteria. *World J Diabetes* 2015; 6:234–44.

7. National Institute for Health and Care Excellence. Diabetes in pregnancy: management from preconception to the postnatal period: NG3. London: NICE, 2015.

8. Diabetes Prevention Program Research Group. Long term effects of metformin on diabetes prevention: Identification of subgroups that benefited most in the Diabetes Prevention Program and Diabetes Prevention Program Outcomes Study. *Diabetes Care* 2019;42:601–8.

9. Diabetes Prevention Program Research Group. Reduction in the incidence of type 2 diabetes with lifestyle intervention or metformin. *N Engl J Med* 2002;346:393–403.

10. Tuomilehto J, Lindstrom J, Eriksson J et al. Prevention of type 2 diabetes mellitus by changes in lifestyle among subjects with impaired glucose tolerance. *N Engl J Med* 2001;344:1343–50.

11. Lindstrom J, Ilanne-Parikka P, Peltonen M et al. Sustained reduction in the incidence of type 2 diabetes by lifestyle intervention: follow up of the Finnish Diabetes Prevention Study. *Lancet* 2006;368:1673–9.

12. Lindstrom J, Peltonen M, Eriksson JG et al. Improved lifestyle and decreased diabetes risk over 13 years: long-term follow-up of the randomised Finnish Diabetes Prevention Study (DPS). *Diabetologia* 2013;56:284–93.

13. Diabetes Prevention Program Research Group. Long-term effects of lifestyle intervention or metformin on diabetes development and microvascular complications over 15 year follow-up: the Diabetes Prevention Program Outcomes Study. *Lancet Diabetes Endocrinol* 2015;3:866–75.

14. Sussman JB, Kent DM, Nelson JP, Hayward RA. Improving diabetes prevention with benefit based tailored treatment: risk based reanalysis of Diabetes Prevention Program. *BMJ* 2015;350:h454.

15. Diabetes Prevention Program Research Group. HbA1c as a predictor of diabetes and as an outcome in the Diabetes Prevention Program: A randomized clinical trial. *Diabetes Care* 2015;38:51–8.

16. Barry E, Roberts S, Oke J et al. Efficacy and effectiveness of screen and treat policies in prevention of type 2 diabetes: systematic review and meta-analysis of screening tests and interventions. *BMJ* 2017;356.

17. Li G, Zhang P, Wang J et al. Cardiovascular mortality, all-cause mortality and diabetes incidence after lifestyle intervention for people with impaired glucose tolerance in the Da Qing Diabetes Prevention Study: a 23 year follow up study. *Lancet Diabetes Endocrinol* 2014;2:474–80.

18. Wareham N. The long-term benefits of lifestyle interventions for prevention of diabetes. *Lancet Diabetes Endocrinol* 2014;2:441–2.

19. Public Health England. A systematic review and meta-analysis assessing effectiveness of pragmatic lifestyle interventions for the prevention of type 2 diabetes in routine practice. London: Public Health England, 2015.

Further resource: information leaflet

WAKEUP Study Group. So you have pre-diabetes? https://medicine.exeter.ac.uk/media/universityofexeter/medicalschool/research/healthservicesresearch/docs/primarycare/WAKEUP_Pre-diabetes_patient_booklet_9-2-16_Read_or_Print.pdf, last accessed 3 July 2020.

3 Diagnosis

In contrast to individuals with type 1 diabetes, who are generally very unwell at presentation with symptoms of polyuria, polydipsia and acute weight loss, most people with type 2 diabetes are asymptomatic at diagnosis. Type 2 diabetes is usually identified with routine or opportunistic screening, though some individuals present with symptoms requiring a clinical history, physical examination and confirmatory blood test.

Clinical presentation

Main symptoms at presentation are usually the classic triad of:

- polyuria
- polydipsia
- weight loss.

Polyuria is an increase in volume and passage frequency of urine. It may increase from a normal level of 0.8–2 L in 24 hours to more than 3 L. The urine is usually of pale color.

Polydipsia is excessive thirst, which arises from the dehydration resulting from loss of fluid and electrolytes in the urine.

Weight loss is a consequence of energy loss from glucose remaining in the urine.

Other symptoms may have gradual onset.

Weakness and fatigue are a consequence of dehydration from polyuria and glucosuria (loss of glucose in urine).

Polyphagia. Individuals may report being hungry between meals.

Vision may be affected.

Pruritus vulvae (genital itching) in women or balanitis (inflammation of the prepuce) in men can occur, as fungal infections arise more frequently in the presence of high glucose.

Delayed healing. Prolonged hyperglycemia can lead to immune suppression, affect the microcirculation and cause neuropathy, all of which can contribute to poor wound healing.

Eruptive xanthomas appear as sudden skin eruptions of crops of pink papules (firm pea-sized bumps) with a creamy center. They may appear on the hands, feet, arms, legs and buttocks. The papules may be pruritic (itchy). Eruptive xanthoma occurs as a consequence of high concentrations of plasma triglyceride, as happens with uncontrolled diabetes, but is a very rare finding.

Acanthosis nigricans is a dark patch of skin with a thick velvety texture. It usually appears in the armpits, neck, elbows, knees, knuckles or groin. The affected areas of skin may also itch or smell. High blood levels of insulin trigger epidermal skin cells to reproduce rapidly – the dark patches are a sign of insulin resistance.

In children a diagnosis of type 1 diabetes should always be considered if any symptom is present, and it is the most likely diagnosis even if the child is asymptomatic (see chapter 9). An immediate point-of-care finger prick glucose test may be helpful for children and young people.

Emergency state. Hyperglycemic hyperosmolar state (HHS) can occur in type 2 diabetes if glucose levels become very high. It may present as coma and carries high mortality if not managed rapidly.

Medical history
The initial baseline assessment of an individual with suspected type 2 diabetes requires a comprehensive review of illnesses, medications, family health history, lifestyle and risk factors (Table 3.1).

Laboratory tests
Note that children, young people and anyone with possible type 1 diabetes should have an urgent laboratory measurement of glucose and not glycosylated hemoglobin (HbA1c). HbA1c is not a good guide when glucose levels are changing rapidly (see Table 2.3, page 19).[1,2]

Blood tests. Glucose tests are summarized in chapter 2 (see Table 2.4, page 20). A random plasma glucose of at least 11.1 mmol/L is also diagnostic.[3]

TABLE 3.1

Key features of medical history

- Illnesses: current symptoms and when they began
- Results of any previous blood or urine glucose tests
- History of any diabetic complications
  - Macrovascular (heart, arteries, stroke)
  - Microvascular (eyes, kidneys, nerves)
  - Infections or poor wound healing
  - Periodontal disease
- Medications: all medicines currently taken
- Family history
- Lifestyle: to gauge the level of understanding for appropriate educational materials
- Physical assessment: initial examination focuses on signs of any health problems as well as developing diabetic complications; it should include:
  - height, weight and calculation of BMI
  - blood pressure, including the response to standing (orthostatic measurement) when autonomic dysfunction is suspected
  - funduscopic eye examination
  - examination for acanthosis nigricans and other stigmata of diabetes, such as necrobiosis lipoidica diabeticorum*
  - respiratory examination for fluid overload
  - abdominal examination for enlarged liver or ascites
  - skin examination for poorly healing injuries and signs of reduced circulation
  - foot examination, including palpation of pulses and tests of sensation (proprioception, vibration, light touch) using a monofilament and tuning fork, and reflexes, along with signs of any foot ulceration (see chapter 7)
  - cardiovascular system for signs of heart failure

*A rare skin condition in which lesions normally develop on the lower part of the leg, though other body parts can be affected. It results from collagen degeneration and inflammation associated with the thickening of blood vessel walls and fat deposition. BMI, body mass index.

To assess for diabetic complications, baseline values are needed for:

- fasting lipids (total cholesterol, low-density lipoprotein [LDL]-cholesterol, high-density lipoprotein [HDL]-cholesterol, non-HDL-cholesterol and triglycerides)
- liver function tests
- kidney function tests (serum creatinine and estimated glomerular filtration rate).

Urine tests. Dipstick testing is no longer used to diagnose diabetes – a blood test should always be used.

First-pass urine for measurement of albumin to creatinine ratio (ACR) is also needed, as an elevated ACR is an early indicator of diabetic nephropathy.

Near-patient blood ketone testing may suggest ketoacidosis; a positive result warrants further investigation. The following triad is diagnostic for diabetic ketoacidosis: blood ketones above 3 mmol/L or significant ketonuria; blood glucose over 11 mmol/L or known diabetes; and plasma bicarbonate below 15 mmol/L and/or venous pH below 7.3.[4]

Further tests may need to be requested to differentiate type 2 diabetes from other types (Table 3.2). Correct diagnosis of the type of diabetes is critical for selecting the most appropriate therapy. However, these are specialist tests that take some time to be reported (a diagnosis of type 1 diabetes should never be delayed while awaiting the results).

C-peptide levels may be helpful where it is not possible to differentiate between type 1 and 2 diabetes.

Diabetes-related autoantibodies. Most people with new-onset type 1 diabetes test positive for at least one diabetes-related autoantibody: islet cell cytoplasmic autoantibodies (ICA); glutamic acid decarboxylase autoantibodies (GADA); insulinoma-associated-2 autoantibodies (IA-2A); and/or insulin autoantibodies (IAA). Consequently, this testing can help to establish a diagnosis of type 1 diabetes or latent autoimmune diabetes in adults (LADA). A negative test does not rule out type 1 diabetes or LADA, however, as some people never develop measurable quantities of these autoantibodies.

Genetic testing. For diagnosing maturity-onset diabetes of the young (MODY), specific genetic testing is required, along with information from clinical and other risk calculators.

TABLE 3.2

Differentiating types of diabetes

Feature	T1DM	LADA	T2DM	MODY
Typical age at onset	Child, though can occur at any age	>30 years	Adult	<25 years
Proportion of all diabetes	~8%	NR	~90%	1–2%
Typical appearance	Normal/thin	Normal/ overweight	Overweight/ obese	Normal
Ethnicity	All	All	All	All
Insulin resistance?	Mostly no (yes in ~10%)	Some	Yes	Depends on type
Presence of autoantibodies?	Yes	Yes in some (mostly GADA), but not in all	Yes in some (GADA present in ~5%)	No
C-peptide levels at diagnosis	Undetectable or extremely low	Low	Normal to high	Depends on type
Ketoacidosis?	Yes	Yes, many not all	Rare	Rare
Insulin secretion	Low/nil	Varies	Varies	Varies

GADA, glutamic acid decarboxylase autoantibodies; LADA, latent autoimmune diabetes in adults; MODY, maturity-onset diabetes of the young; NR, not reported; T1 or T2 DM, type 1 or 2 diabetes mellitus.

Key points – diagnosis

- Type 2 diabetes is usually identified with routine or opportunistic screening, unlike type 1 diabetes.
- Do not use glycosylated hemoglobin (HbA1c) for children, young people, those for whom type 1 diabetes is a possibility or individuals whose glucose levels may be changing over a short period.
- A comprehensive medical history is important; further tests may be necessary to ensure the correct diabetes type is identified.

References

1. World Health Organization. Use of glycated haemoglobin (HbA1c) in the diagnosis of diabetes mellitus. Geneva: WHO, 2011.

2. John WG on behalf of the UK Department of Health Advisory Committee on Diabetes. Use of haemoglobin A1c (HbA1c) in the diagnosis of diabetes mellitus. The implementation of World Health Organization (WHO) guidance 2011. *Diabet Med* 2012;29:1350–7.

3. American Diabetes Association. 2. Classification and Diagnosis of Diabetes: Standards of Medical Care in Diabetes—2020. *Diabetes Care* 2020;43(Suppl 1): S14–31.

4. Kohler K, Levy N. Management of diabetic ketoacidosis: a summary of the 2013 Joint British Diabetes Societies guidelines. *J Intensive Care Soc* 2014;15:222–5.

4 Self-management

The charity Diabetes UK estimates people with diabetes spend 2–3 hours each year interacting with health professionals and self-manage their diabetes for 8758 hours. Patient-centered care is a central theme in diabetes, supported by the National Institute for Health and Care Excellence (NICE),[1] the Scottish Intercollegiate Guidelines Network (SIGN)[2] and the American Diabetes Association (ADA)/ European Association for the Study of Diabetes (EASD) 2018 consensus statement.[3] Clinicians should strive to share enough information to allow people with diabetes to feel empowered (or activated) and in control of their own decisions, as this can help them achieve better outcomes.[4]

It can take 18–24 months for people to understand their diabetes and how to manage it. More information-sharing is needed in the early stages; for some people, information-gathering about how they want to manage their diabetes is needed at later stages. Getting that balance right can be tricky. Health professionals should continue to reflect on whether they are being too didactic and need to allow more autonomy, particularly around adherence, medication choices and inertia.

Key concepts
Diabetes self-management can be challenging and confusing. Effective information and support should help to equip people to safely manage their type 2 diabetes in an autonomous way.

Empowerment and health literacy. The World Health Organization has defined patient empowerment as 'A process in which patients understand their role, are given the knowledge and skills by their healthcare provider to perform a task in an environment that recognizes community and cultural differences and encourages patient participation.'[5] Messages need to be delivered in a way that recognizes the person's cultural background and level of understanding (health literacy). Health literacy – 'a measure of patients' ability to read, comprehend, and act on medical instructions' – varies considerably and this needs to be taken into account in discussions and when supplying written information.

Language use, particularly in early conversations with people about diabetes diagnosis, can be very impactful in helping people have a positive (or negative) attitude to their diabetes. The NHS England resource *Language Matters* has more information on this and has been produced to support communication with people with diabetes.[6]

Psychological impact. Several factors can have a psychological impact around diagnosis: the permanency of diabetes; guilt and self-blame; shame; stigma; fear; lack of understanding; the realization of the need to make changes and take medication; and thoughts of friends and family who have not fared well with diabetes. This psychological effect can lead to diabetes-related distress and depression, a risk that persists throughout the disease course and may negatively impact on outcomes.

At diagnosis, people need time and support to adjust to the diagnosis. Around one-third of individuals adjust well, one-third have problems and need support and one-third struggle to make adjustments. Older people, vulnerable groups, those with low health literacy, comorbidities and poor social support may need more support.

Behavior change and motivational interviewing

Many behavior changes are recommended to people with type 2 diabetes, often while they are still coming to terms with the diagnosis. Changing behavior can be difficult. Reflecting on our own health behaviors reminds us how difficult it can be to achieve lasting changes. Using tools such as motivational interviewing can empower people to take action.

The stages of change model (Figure 4.1) is a simple way to understand whether people are ready to make changes. Listening closely when asking questions such as 'What do you think about losing weight?' or 'What do you think about making changes to your diet?' helps us understand the stage of change the individual is at and

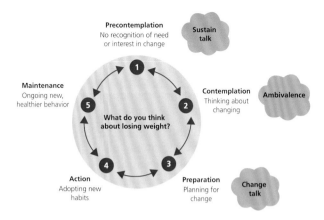

Figure 4.1 Recognizing stages of change.

therefore the type of guidance to offer. If their response focuses on why change is impossible, so-called 'sustain talk', it suggests they are in the precontemplation stage. Responding with equal discussion of pros and cons about making the change suggests they are in the contemplation stage and facing ambivalence. In both these stages, offering advice about lifestyle changes is unhelpful, as the individual is not ready to change. Instead, helping the person to identify personal advantages to changing may move them toward the preparation stage. When positive or 'change talk' is obvious, it is likely they are in the preparation stage and may welcome advice if offered.

Motivational interviewing is a consultation style that seeks to harness the person's own motivation and help resolve ambivalence, so he or she is more likely to choose to take action to make lifestyle changes.

Motivational interviewing models usually have four (overlapping) stages, which often have different names:
- building rapport – active listening, empathy, non-verbal skills, open questions, affirmations, summarizing
- setting a shared agenda
- establishing importance – understanding why making the change is important to the person
- exploring and enhancing confidence – eliciting barriers, encouraging problem solving.

Health professionals inherently use some motivational interviewing skills. Building on this with additional skills can enhance satisfaction and outcomes when discussing any behavior change, but these are best learned face-to-face from experts.

Most health professionals are skilled at building rapport. Letting people set the agenda for the lifestyle consultation by using a balloon or bubble diagram (Figure 4.2) improves empowerment. If there are pressing matters to discuss – such as changes to treatment – seek permission to add these to the shared agenda.

Using importance and confidence rulers can help identify why a specific behavior change is important to the individual and how confident they feel to achieve it, opening up discussion. 'On a scale of 1–10, with 10 at the top, how important is it to you to lose weight?' Asking 'Why is it a 9 and not a 5?' leads to discussion and more information. Encourage people to express the personal, positive, emotional benefits of taking action so they persuade and motivate themselves to choose to change. Capture their reasons for future discussions.

Recognizing someone is still in precontemplation (expressing more sustain talk, see Figure 4.1, page 39), it may be appropriate, with permission, to share potential benefits. The more we listen for change and sustain talk, the better we get at hearing it and accurately identifying the stage of change.

'On a scale of 1–10, how confident are you that you could lose weight?' Asking 'Why is it a 5 and not a 2?' allows exploration of why

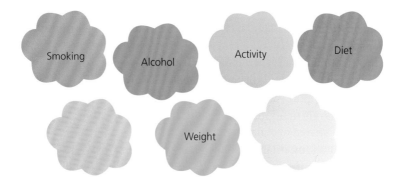

Figure 4.2 Using a bubble or balloon diagram to facilitate lifestyle discussions.

they believe they could achieve the change. 'What would it take to move you to an 8?' helps identify barriers and facilitates action-planning and shared decision-making.

Despite little evidence that motivational interviewing specifically improves glycemic management,[7] it remains a useful tool to help people motivate themselves to make lifestyle or other changes.

What self-management options do people *want* to discuss? As the majority of people with type 2 diabetes will die from cardiovascular disease (CVD), we tend to deliver self-management education that focuses on helping them reduce cardiovascular risk factors, such as smoking and excessive alcohol intake, and adhere to medication. As there is extensive information available elsewhere about diet, physical activity and smoking cessation, the next section focuses on signposting to useful resources.

Lifestyle advice
Weight management. Everyone should be encouraged to move toward achieving and maintaining a healthy weight. In prevention studies, progression from non-diabetic hyperglycemia (NDH) to type 2 diabetes was reduced significantly by weight loss of 5–7 kg; in DiRECT (the DIabetes REmission Clinical Trial), involving people with less than 6 years' duration of type 2 diabetes, more than 80% of those who managed to lose more than 15 kg (on an 825 kcal diet) achieved remission at 12 months, with significant remission also in those losing more than 10 kg.[8]

Goal setting. Encourage people to be realistic when goal setting, aiming for an initial 2–3 kg weight loss and to set specific, measured, action-oriented, realistic and timed (SMART) goals.

Individualizing diet and lifestyle advice. There is no single diet that suits everyone and if the eating pattern adopted is chosen by the individual and fits their lifestyle, it is more likely to be sustainable. Eating carbohydrates stimulates insulin release, triggering increased fat storage. There is no evidence that low-fat diets reduce CVD risk. Recommendations are slowly changing. Diabetes UK's 'Evidence-based nutrition guidelines for the prevention and management of diabetes'[9] and the ADA nutrition guideline[10] reflect this change in thinking. They provide summaries of eating patterns and their evidence, and they include guidance for those with type 2 diabetes and CVD or chronic kidney disease (CKD). The Mediterranean diet (relatively low in carbohydrates and high in 'good' fats such as nuts, olive oil and avocados) is effective in helping people lose weight, improve glycemic control and reduce the risk of first and subsequent CVD events. Simple messages such as portion control with pictures may suit those with low health literacy. The ADA guideline highlights the evidence base for low-carbohydrate diets.

Sugar-sweetened beverages. Encourage a reduction in the intake of sugar-sweetened beverages; if the person is drinking significant quantities, changing to those containing non-nutritive sweeteners (NNS) in the short term and in moderation may help weight loss.[4] However, some studies demonstrate NNS cause weight gain, and the 2020 ADA Standards of Medical Care[4] recommend avoiding these too and replacing with water.

Alcohol. The recommended maximum number of weekly units in the UK is 14. There is no evidence that small amounts of alcohol are harmful in diabetes, but an excess can increase the risks of hypoglycemia, weight gain and poor glycemic control.

Physical activity. A summary of physical activity recommendations is shown in Table 4.1; more detailed guidance is provided in the SIGN management guidelines.[2] The 2016 ADA guidelines provide more detailed physical activity recommendations, including recommendations for those with complications and for those using insulin.[11]

Smoking cessation. Smokers with diabetes (and passive smokers) have increased risks of CVD, premature death and microvascular complications and worse glycemic control when compared with non-smokers. Encourage people to stop smoking. Smoking cessation can lead to weight gain. For those without type 2 diabetes, this increases the risk of developing it for several years after cessation; however, the CVD benefit outweighs this risk. The increase in risk does not occur if weight gain is avoided. In newly diagnosed people with type 2 diabetes and albuminuria, smoking cessation reduces the risk of albuminuria progression as well as having beneficial effects on CVD risk.[12]

TABLE 4.1

Physical activity recommendations

- Decrease sedentary time
- Avoid prolonged sitting – standing up every 30 minutes can improve glycemia
- Aim for 150 minutes of moderate to vigorous physical activity per week (e.g. walking briskly) spread over at least 3 days, with no more than 2 days without activity; 75 minutes of vigorous activity or interval training may be recommended instead for younger and fitter people if preferred
- Aim for 2–3 sessions of resistance exercise per week on non-consecutive days
- Older people should add 2–3 sessions of flexibility and balance training – yoga and tai chi may be suitable
- Individualize recommendations
- Arrange pre-exercise assessment for those with established cardiovascular disease or at high risk before undertaking anything more strenuous than walking
- People with neuropathy and proliferative retinopathy should consult their specialist before undertaking activities other than walking

Source: American Diabetes Association 2019.[4]

A 2014 Cochrane systematic review concluded that studies using electronic cigarettes were small and the results inconsistent.[13] Electronic cigarettes containing nicotine were more effective at aiding smoking cessation and helping reduce the number of cigarettes smoked than those without nicotine. Electronic cigarettes have been demonstrated in one study to be twice as effective at aiding cessation

Practice point

As healthcare practitioners, we should encourage healthier lifestyles at every opportunity. 'Make every contact count' – multiple very brief interventions may be more effective than a single longer one.

as nicotine replacement therapy (NRT), but 80% were still using them at 12 months versus 9% with NRT. The ADA no longer recommends their use as an aid to cessation because of the risk of addiction among young people and health risks linked with vaping.

What information do people with diabetes *need* to stay safe?

People are unlikely to spontaneously ask for this information, so it needs to be offered.

Self-monitoring of blood glucose. Both NICE and SIGN recommend self-monitoring of blood glucose (SMBG) for those on insulin and those who are pregnant or planning pregnancy.[1,2] NICE also recommends SMBG for those who:

- have evidence of hypoglycemia
- are on oral therapy that may increase the risk of hypoglycemia while driving or operating machinery.

SIGN also recommends SMBG be considered in those who are:[2]

- at increased risk of hypoglycemia
- experiencing acute illness
- undergoing significant changes in drug therapy or fasting (e.g. for Ramadan)
- suffering with unstable or poor glycemic control (glycosylated hemoglobin [HbA1c] >64 mmol/mol [8%]).

Consider short-term monitoring when starting oral or intravenous corticosteroids or to confirm suspected hypoglycemia. In those with type 2 diabetes not using insulin, the effects of SMBG on improving control are small but positive.

Those using SMBG should have a structured assessment at least annually, discussing self-monitoring skills, frequency and quality of testing, checking they can interpret the results and use them to take action, the benefits and the impact on quality of life.

Ensure all drivers using insulin report this to the Driver & Vehicle Licensing Agency (DVLA) and that all drivers at risk of hypoglycemia (including those on sulfonylureas, meglitinides and insulin) monitor their levels at times relevant to driving.

Having a second severe hypoglycemic episode (requiring third-party assistance) while awake in a 12-month period must be reported to the DVLA, as must having one severe hypoglycemic attack while driving.

In both instances, the person must stop driving. Consult the DVLA's guidance *Assessing Fitness to Drive* for full up-to-date information on diabetes and driving.[14] Document the advice given in the individual's electronic record.

Hypoglycemia is defined as plasma glucose below 4 mmol/L (<3.9 mmol/L in the USA) and should be treated. Severe hypoglycemia occurs when assistance from a third party (family member, friend, paramedic) is required to help treat the hypoglycemia. The true prevalence of hypoglycemia is unknown as people tend to under-report it, particularly drivers who are aware of the regulations around driving and severe daytime hypoglycemia.

Insulin-treated people have, on average, two mild hypoglycemic episodes per week and up to two serious events per year. For those with type 2 diabetes treated with sulfonylureas, the risk of hypoglycemia is 2.5–3 times higher than for those using metformin. Severe hypoglycemia can cause permanent neurological deficit. Mortality is 3–4 times higher in the years following a severe hypoglycemic episode than among those with mild hypoglycemia; there is a 22% mortality risk within 12 months in those with type 2 diabetes who have a severe hypoglycemic episode. Ensuing fear can have a significant impact on self-management. We should be aware that people are likely to avoid future hypoglycemia by keeping blood sugar high through non-adherence to medication.

TABLE 4.2

Signs and symptoms of hypoglycemia

Adrenergic (activation of the sympathetic nervous system)	Neuroglycopenic (brain glucose deprivation)
• Sweating	• Slurred speech
• Shaking	• Unusual behavior
• Palpitations	• Poor coordination
• Feeling hungry	• Confusion
• Tingling	• Drowsiness
• Headache and nausea	• Coma

TABLE 4.3

Management of hypoglycemia

- 15–20 g fast-acting carbohydrate if conscious and able to swallow
  - 5–6 dextrose tablets
  - 5 large jelly babies
  - 7 large jelly beans
  - 200 mL (small carton) smooth orange juice
  - Lucozade, 170–220 mL*
  - 2 tubes of 40% glucose gel
- Wait 15 minutes and retest
- If plasma glucose still <4 mmol/L, or not feeling better, repeat the treatment up to twice more
- If unconscious or unable to swallow, do not give anything by mouth; place in the recovery position and call an ambulance; give glucagon if available
- Once the person is feeling better, encourage him or her to either proceed with a meal or eat a small snack containing carbohydrate (e.g. sandwich, two plain biscuits or a banana)
- If taking a sulfonylurea, either arrange for careful monitoring for 24 hours or admit, as further hypoglycemia may occur

*Lucozade has been reformulated with 50% less sugar, so 100 mL is no longer enough.

Common causes include delayed or missed meals, eating less carbohydrate, drinking alcohol or increased activity. People with cognitive problems, CKD, hypoglycemia unawareness or autonomic neuropathy are at increased risk, as are pregnant women aiming for tight glucose control.

Advice. People at risk of hypoglycemia should be counseled about signs and symptoms (Table 4.2) and management (Table 4.3) at every consultation. Ensure access to SMBG and encourage testing whenever symptoms develop. Many people fail to test when they are hypoglycemic and do not carry treatment with them.

Older people experience adrenergic signs and symptoms at lower glucose levels, are more likely to develop neuroglycopenic symptoms before they can take action and are therefore more likely to develop severe hypoglycemia (needing assistance from a third party). Falls and fractures can result in older people and decrease independence. More detail is available in the TREND-UK guideline,[15] which can be shared with care home staff and other members of the health team.

After severe hypoglycemia, it is important to arrange a medication review, including consideration of decreasing the insulin dose by 10–20%.

Frequent hypoglycemia and autonomic neuropathy can result in decreased or absent hypoglycemia awareness, greatly increasing the risk of severe hypoglycemia, which can occur without warning signs or symptoms. Sometimes this can be improved by changing therapy or completely avoiding hypoglycemia for prolonged periods. Referral to the specialist team is appropriate.

Sick day guidance. When people with type 2 diabetes suffer an intercurrent illness, they need to understand how to keep themselves safe (Table 4.4). If they are at risk of dehydration (from diarrhea and vomiting), they need to pause/stop drugs that may cause acute kidney injury or hypoglycemia – the 'SADMAN' rules are given in Table 4.5. Advise the person to restart these drugs once they are eating and drinking normally. NHS Scotland provides cards which can be personalized to remind the person which drugs to stop when at risk of dehydration.

Remind people with type 2 diabetes to continue with other treatments when they are ill, and that infections and other conditions can cause blood sugar to rise, even when not eating. This can be hard to understand and people often stop medication, including insulin, precipitating ketoacidosis or hyperosmolar hyperglycemia (especially in frail older people) that requires urgent admission.

More detailed information on how to manage insulin during illness is available in 'How to advise on sick day rules'.[16]

Self-management education

Self-management education should be delivered at the time of diagnosis, annually, when complications arise, at times of transition and, ideally, at every opportunity ('make every contact count').

TABLE 4.4

General advice for managing diabetes during illness

S (Sugar)	• Blood sugar levels can rise during illness even if not eating
	• Those with access to blood glucose monitoring should increase testing frequency
I (Insulin)	• People should understand NEVER to stop their insulin or other medication, apart from the specific medications listed in Table 4.5
	• Insulin doses may need to be increased (see the guidance below for detailed advice); recommend patients speak to their diabetes specialist nurse the same day for advice
C (Carbohydrates)	• Ensure hydration and carbohydrate intake continue
	• If unable to eat or vomiting, replace food with sugary drinks
	• If plasma glucose levels are high, use sugar-free fluids to maintain hydration
	• If plasma glucose levels are low, encourage regular intake of sugary drinks
K (Ketones)	• Are mainly of concern in those with type 1 diabetes; drink plenty water to maintain hydration
	• Test ketones every 2–4 hours and discuss results with diabetes specialist nurse or GP

Source: Down 2018.[16]

Self-management education can occur at three levels:
- information and one-to-one advice offered during consultations (e.g. Diabetes UK information prescriptions or booklets, DVLA guidance on driving)
- ongoing informal education (e.g. My Diabetes and Me, Pocket Medic diabetes videos)
- formal structured education programs.

Diabetes UK has collated information on other resources that may be helpful.[17] 'Learning Zone' is a free to use e-learning course developed by Diabetes UK. Information prescriptions can be embedded in practice software and personalized and printed out during consultations.

Structured education programs. NICE states that people should be offered a structured education program at diagnosis. Numbers referred to and attending structured education are captured in the National Diabetes Audit.

To meet NICE criteria, structured education programs must:[1,18]

- be tailored to the individual
- be evidence-based, with specific aims and learning objectives
- support people with diabetes and their carers to develop beliefs, attitudes, knowledge and skills to self-manage diabetes
- have a structured, evidence-based, theory-driven curriculum with supporting materials
- be delivered by appropriately trained educators
- be quality assured, with review by independent assessors against standard criteria to ensure consistency
- have outcomes audited regularly.

TABLE 4.5

SADMAN guidance: drugs to stop when at risk of dehydration

S	SGLT2 inhibitors	Increased risk of euglycemic DKA
A	ACE inhibitors	Increased risk of AKI if dehydrated
D	Diuretics	Increased risk of AKI if dehydrated
M	Metformin	Increased risk of developing lactic acidosis (rare)
A	ARBs	Increased risk of AKI if dehydrated
N	NSAIDs	Increased risk of AKI due to reduced afferent vasodilatation

ACE, angiotensin-converting enzyme; AKI, acute kidney injury; ARB angiotensin II receptor blocker; DKA, diabetic ketoacidosis; NSAID, non-steroidal anti-inflammatory drug; SGLT2, sodium–glucose cotransporter 2.

In addition, they should meet the cultural, linguistic, cognitive and literacy levels of the group. Other forms of education should be available for those unable to attend a structured education program.

DESMOND and X-PERT programs are available across the UK, as are locally developed programs (DESMOND is Diabetes Education and Self-Management for Ongoing and Newly Diagnosed). These programs aim to provide knowledge and skills.

A cluster randomized controlled trial of DESMOND demonstrated weight loss, reduced smoking, a positive change in illness beliefs and reduced depression score in program participants at 12 months, but no significant HbA1c decrease compared with controls (0.4%).[19] When the overall benefits of small changes in multiple risk factors are considered, DESMOND is likely to be cost-effective compared with normal care, with reductions in weight and smoking being the main benefits delivered.[20]

A randomized controlled trial that compared the X-PERT program with one-to-one consultations with a dietitian demonstrated 82% attendance for at least four of six X-PERT sessions.[21] The X-PERT group achieved a significant 0.6% reduction in HbA1c, and significant reductions in weight, BMI, waist circumference and total cholesterol, a reduction in medication requirement and increases in fruit and vegetable consumption, physical activity and foot care. Program participants had improved food enjoyment, greater treatment satisfaction, increased diabetes knowledge and greater self-empowerment.

Attendance at structured education programs is very low and SIGN has advocated computer-assisted education packages such as 'My Diabetes and Me'. A recent UK study of reasons for declining structured education found multiple disparate reasons, suggesting there is no single solution to increasing attendance.[22] Many individuals felt they knew enough to manage their diabetes, but this was not supported by testing essential diabetes self-management knowledge.

User-friendly education resources available online have been developed across the UK. In Wales, Pocket Medic videos can be prescribed. Each one provides a short, professionally produced, audio-visual discussion about one specific aspect of diabetes. These have been validated as improving information delivery.

Key points – self-management

- People with type 2 diabetes spend around 2 hours per year with a healthcare professional and 8758 hours managing their disease themselves. Self-management skills are therefore important.
- Consider patient empowerment, health literacy, positive language and diabetes distress and depression when looking after people with type 2 diabetes.
- Self-monitoring of blood glucose should be available for those at risk of hypoglycemia and/or using insulin and for women who are pregnant or planning a pregnancy.
- Building motivational interviewing or its tools into behavior-change consultations improves outcomes.
- Discuss weight, activity and smoking cessation at every opportunity.
- Ensure people at risk of hypoglycemia and carers know how to manage hypoglycemia and when to get help.
- Ensure people with type 2 diabetes know which drugs to temporarily stop when at risk of dehydration and when to restart them.
- Encourage all people newly diagnosed with type 2 diabetes to attend a local structured education program.

References

1. National Institute for Health and Care Excellence. Type 2 diabetes in adults: management: NG28. London: NICE, 2015.

2. Scottish Intercollegiate Guidelines Network. Management of diabetes. Edinburgh: SIGN, 2010, updated 2017.

3. Davies M, D'Alessio D, Fradkin J et al. Management of hyperglycemia in type 2 diabetes, 2018. A consensus report by the American Diabetes Association (ADA) and the European Association for the Study of Diabetes (EASD). *Diabetes Care* 2018;41: 2669–701.

4. American DIabetes Association. 5. Facilitating behavior change and well-being to improve health outcomes: Standards of medical care in diabetes—2020. *Diabetes Care* 2020;43(Suppl 1):S48–65.

5. World Health Organization. 2 Patient empowerment and health care. In: *WHO Guidelines on Hand Hygiene in Health Care: First Global Patient Safety Challenge Clean Care is Safer Care*. Geneva: World Health Organization, 2009. www.ncbi.nlm.nih.gov/books/NBK144022, last accessed 3 July 2020.

6. NHS England. Language matters: language and diabetes. 2018. www.england.nhs.uk/publication/language-matters-language-and-diabetes, last accessed 3 July 2020.

7. Rosenbek Minet LK, Wagner L, Lønvig EM, et al. The effect of motivational interviewing on glycaemic control and perceived competence of diabetes self-management in patients with type 1 and type 2 diabetes mellitus after attending a group education programme: a randomised controlled trial. *Diabetologia* 2011;54:1620–9.

8. Lean M, Leslie W, Barnes A, et al. Primary care-led weight management for remission of type 2 diabetes (DiRECT): an open-label cluster-randomised trial. *Lancet* 2017;391:541–51.

9. Dyson PA, Twenefour D, Breen C et al. Diabetes UK evidence-based nutrition guidelines for the prevention and management of diabetes. *Diabet Med* 2018;35:541–7.

10. Evert AB, Dennison M, Gardner C et al. Nutrition therapy for adults with diabetes or prediabetes: a consensus report. *Diabetes Care* 2019;42:731–54.

11. Colberg SR, Sigal RJ, Yardley JE et al. Physical activity/exercise and diabetes: a position statement of the American Diabetes Association. *Diabetes Care* 2016;39:2065–79.

12. Voulgari C, Katsilambros N, Tentolouris N. Smoking cessation predicts amelioration of microalbuminuria in newly diagnosed type 2 diabetes mellitus: a 1 year prospective study. *Metabolism* 2011;60:1456–64.

13. McRobbie H, Bullen C, Hartmann-Boyce J, Hajek P. Electronic cigarettes for smoking cessation and reduction. *Cochrane Database Syst Rev* 2014:CD010216.

14. Driver & Vehicle Licensing Agency. Assessing fitness to drive – a guide for medical professionals. London: Department for Transport, 2019. www.gov.uk/government/publications/assessing-fitness-to-drive-a-guide-for-medical-professionals, last accessed 3 July 2020.

15. Hicks D, Hill J, James J. For healthcare professionals: hypoglycaemia in adults in the community: recognition, management and prevention. TREND-UK, 2019. https://trend-uk.org/portfolio/hypoglycaemia-in-adults-in-the-community-recognition-management-and-prevention, last accessed 3 July 2020.

16. Down S. How to advise on sick day rules. *Diabetes & Primary Care* 2018;20:15-16.

17. Diabetes UK. Diabetes self-management education. www.diabetes.org.uk/professionals/resources/resources-to-improve-your-clinical-practice/diabetes-self-management-education, last accessed 3 July 2020.

18. National Institute for Health and Care Excellence. Diabetes in adults: QS6. London: NICE, 2011, updated 2016.

19. Davies MJ, Heller S, Skinner TC et al. Effectiveness of the diabetes education and self management for ongoing and newly diagnosed (DESMOND) programme for people with newly diagnosed type 2 diabetes: cluster randomised controlled trial. *BMJ* 2008;336:491–5.

20. Gillett M, Dallosso HM, Dixon S et al. Delivering diabetes education and self management for people with newly diagnosed type 2 diabetes: cost effectiveness analysis. *BMJ* 2010;341:c4093.

21. Deakin TA, Cade JE, Williams R, Greenwood DC. Structured patient education: the Diabetes X-PERT programme makes a difference. *Diab Med* 2006;23:944–54.

22. Coates V, Slevin M, Carey M et al. Declining structured diabetes education in those with type 2 diabetes: a plethora of individual and organisational reasons. *Patient Educ Couns* 2018;101:696–702.

Further resource: sick day rules card/leaflet

Healthcare Improvement Scotland/ Scottish Patient Safety Programme. Medicines sick day rules card. https:// ihub.scot/improvement-programmes/ scottish-patient-safety-programme- spsp/spsp-medicines-collaborative/ high-risk-situations-involving- medicines/medicines-sick-day-rules- card/, last accessed 3 July 2020.

5

Lowering blood glucose

Although this chapter focuses initially on glycemic control, multifactorial intervention – including blood pressure and lipid management, smoking cessation, weight management, diet and exercise – from the time of diagnosis maximizes benefits. Guidelines in common use in the UK are shown in Useful Resources, page 146. All the guidelines stress the importance of patient-centered care, individualization of targets and avoiding clinical inertia.

The Scottish Intercollegiate Guidelines Network (SIGN) guideline and American Diabetes Association (ADA)/European Association for the Study of Diabetes (EASD) consensus statement (2018, updated in 2019) take account of new evidence from cardiovascular outcome trials (CVOTs) and specify that people with established cardiovascular disease (CVD) or at high risk of CVD, or with heart failure or chronic kidney disease (CKD) should be offered drugs demonstrated to decrease mortality, morbidity or CKD progression.[1-3] At the time of writing, the National Institute for Health and Care Excellence (NICE) is updating its guidelines.

NICE Medicines Optimisation Priorities, updated annually, offer guidance on maintaining or improving the quality of medicines use. Key therapeutic topics include type 2 diabetes, safer insulin prescribing, multimorbidity and polypharmacy, and shared decision-making.[4]

Achieving glycemic control

The key tasks in achieving glycemic control are shown in Table 5.1. Multifactorial risk management is required, including lifestyle, glycemic control, and blood pressure and lipid management. Do not focus solely on glycemia. Blood pressure and lipid management are covered in chapter 6.

Agree an individualized glycemic target. Follow a structured approach to agreeing the glycemic target and discussing drug therapy with the individual. The glycemic target should take into account the

TABLE 5.1

Key tasks to achieve glycemic control

- Agree an individualized glycemic target
- Counsel on diet and lifestyle and encourage lifestyle change
- Initiate medication – metformin first line unless contraindicated
- Intensify therapy to achieve individualized target, taking account of CVD, CKD, heart failure, need to manage weight, need to avoid hypoglycemia, and cost/cost-effectiveness
- Initiate injectable therapy with GLP-1RA or insulin if needed

CKD, chronic kidney disease; CVD, cardiovascular disease;
GLP-1RA, glucagon-like peptide-1 receptor agonist.

person's needs, circumstances, preferences and comorbidities as well as risks from hypoglycemia and polypharmacy. Once the target is agreed, help the person achieve it safely by rechecking their glycosylated hemoglobin (HbA1c) level 3 months after each therapy change. Avoid clinical inertia – failing to intensify therapy to meet agreed glycemic or other goals – which is commonplace.

Figure 5.1 aims to help clinicians to individualize glycemic targets. NICE has developed a decision aid to help people with type 2 diabetes choose a glycemic target and make medication choices after metformin.[5]

Early tight glycemic control initiated soon after diagnosis reduces microvascular and possibly macrovascular complications and provides a long-lasting 'legacy effect'.[6] Tight glycemic control late in the disease course is more difficult to achieve and may be harmful.

NICE has recommended glycemic targets, which can then be individualized:[7]

- HbA1c of 48 mmol/mol (6.5%) or lower for those on lifestyle intervention or metformin or other initial drug therapy (that does not cause hypoglycemia)
- HbA1c of 53 mmol/mol (7.0%) or lower for those on a sulfonylurea, and at first and subsequent intensification to dual, triple and injectable therapies.

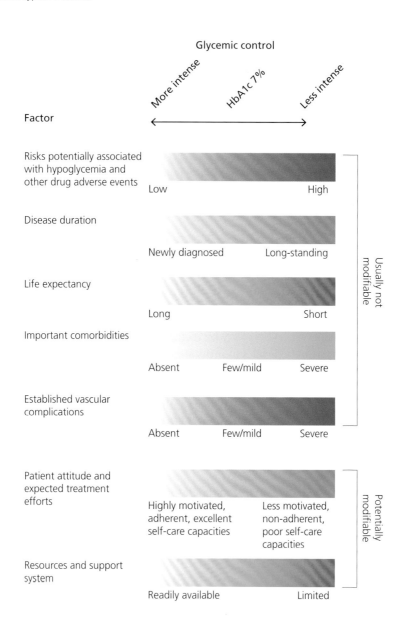

Figure 5.1 Factors to consider when helping people choose a glycemic target. HbA1c, glycosylated hemoglobin. Adapted from Inzucchi et al. 2015.[8]

Practice point

Review the HbA1c values for people with less than 10 years' duration of type 2 diabetes in your practice. Are you helping people achieve tight early glycemic control?

If HbA1c rises to 58 mmol/mol (7.5%) or higher, therapy should be further intensified; assist the individual to achieve an HbA1c of 53 mmol/mol or lower, or their individualized target. These targets also apply for subsequent intensifications, including initiation of insulin if required.

The ADA/EASD consensus statement does not make specific recommendations for glycemic targets, but instead encourages individualization.[2,3] Glycemic targets in older and/or frail people are discussed further in chapter 9 on special populations.

Counsel on diet and lifestyle. If there is scope for significant changes in lifestyle that may result in weight loss and improve glycemic control *and* if the person is motivated to make changes or they are resistant to immediately starting drug therapy, discuss a 3-month trial of lifestyle intervention. Refer the person to a dietitian or to a local exercise on prescription or weight loss service. If HbA1c is high, the individual is symptomatic or there is evidence of complications, consider initiating drug therapy immediately. Counsel the person about the benefits of tight early glycemic control and check HbA1c at 3 months. Short-term sulfonylurea therapy may be needed if symptomatic. The management of blood pressure and lipids is discussed in chapter 6.

Initiate metformin. To minimize gastrointestinal side effects, 'start low and go slow' with dose increases. Initiate 500 mg metformin and encourage the individual to increase at weekly intervals to 1 g twice daily (1 g daily if estimated glomerular filtration rate [eGFR] <45 mL/min/1.73 m²). Gastrointestinal symptoms such as bloating, colicky abdominal pain and diarrhea can be troublesome. If this is the case, advise the person to revert to a lower dose and increase the dose more slowly. Encourage the person to seek further advice if they remain intolerant. Consider switching to modified-release metformin which is, anecdotally, better tolerated. Metformin is not recommended if eGFR is below 30 mL/min/1.73 m².

> **Practice point** (PP)
>
> Ensure the person knows that metformin is long-term therapy.
> Issue an initial acute prescription outlining the dose escalation
> then add a repeat script for metformin at full dose, otherwise there is a
> risk the person will cycle through the doses with each subsequent script
> or no repeat will be issued until he or she is seen again.

Check HbA1c 3 months after taking metformin at the full tolerated
dose. If still above the agreed target, intensify therapy.

Intensify therapy. Consider whether it is helpful to share a decision
aid or leaflet regarding therapy choices. Revisit the agreed glycemic
target. The 2019 ADA/EASD consensus update recommends
considering the addition of glucagon-like peptide-1 receptor agonists
(GLP-1 RAs) or sodium–glucose cotransporter 2 (SGLT2) inhibitors in
those with CVD, CKD or heart failure, even if at glycemic target.[3]
When treatment intensification is considered, discuss lifestyle changes
and check for side effects and adherence with current medication
before adding therapy.

Check whether the individual has established atherosclerotic CVD
(ASCVD), CKD or heart failure or is at high risk of ASCVD. If yes,
follow the updated ADA/EASD consensus statement as follows.[2,3]

If ASCVD predominates or there is a high risk of ASCVD
(see Figure 5.2), discuss and initiate a GLP-1RA with proven CVD
benefit (liraglutide, semaglutide or dulaglutide; there is evidence only
for dulaglutide in those with risk factors) in preference to an SGLT2
inhibitor with proven CVD benefit, if the patient agrees; check HbA1c
after 3 months. If still above target, consider adding an SGLT2
inhibitor or other drugs with proven cardiovascular benefit or safety.

If heart failure or CKD predominates (eGFR < 60 mL/min/1.73 m²
or albuminuria; see Figure 5.3), the consensus recommends we discuss
and initiate an SGLT2 inhibitor with evidence of reducing hospitalization
for heart failure and/or CKD progression (empagliflozin, canagliflozin,
dapagliflozin) if eGFR is adequate (≥60 mL/min/1.73 m² for
dapagliflozin or empagliflozin; canagliflozin can be initiated at lower
eGFR – see summary of product characteristics [SmPC] for details).
If an SGLT2 inhibitor is not tolerated or contraindicated, add a GLP-1RA
with proven CVD benefit (see above). Avoid pioglitazone and

saxagliptin if the person has heart failure. If the person is not using a GLP-1RA, consider adding a dipeptidyl peptidase-4 (DPP-4) inhibitor proven to be well tolerated in individuals with heart failure, such as linagliptin or sitagliptin.

Recheck HbA1c at 3-monthly intervals until the agreed HbA1c target is reached. At that stage, HbA1c can be checked 6 monthly.

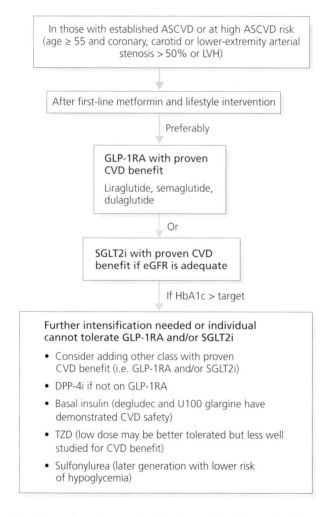

Figure 5.2 Glucose-lowering medication in people with type 2 diabetes and established or at high risk of ASCVD. LVH, left ventricular hypertrophy. See Figure 5.3 for other abbreviations and sources.

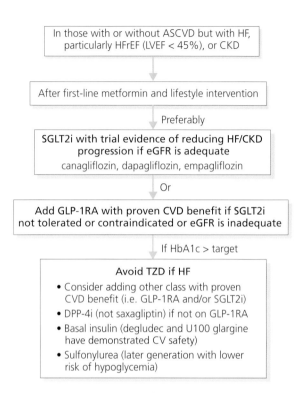

Figure 5.3 Glucose-lowering medication in people with type 2 diabetes where heart failure (HF) or chronic kidney disease (CKD) predominates. ASCVD, atherosclerotic cardiovascular disease; CV(D), cardiovascular (disease); DPP-4i, dipeptidyl peptidase-4 inhibitor; eGFR, estimated glomerular filtration rate; GLP-1RA, glucagon-like peptide-1 receptor agonist; HbA1c, glycosylated hemoglobin; HFrEF, heart failure with reduced ejection fraction; LVEF, left ventricular ejection fraction; SGLT2i, sodium–glucose cotransporter 2 inhibitor; TZD, thiazolidinedione. Adapted from the updated American Diabetes Association/European Association for the Study of Diabetes consensus statement.[2,3]

If there is no ASCVD, heart failure or CKD, consider the therapeutic options on the basis of the most compelling needs:

- minimize hypoglycemia – add DPP-4 inhibitor, GLP-1RA, SGLT2 inhibitor or thiazolidinedione (TZD)
- minimize weight gain or promote weight loss – add GLP-1RA with evidence for weight loss or SGLT2 inhibitor
- keep costs low – add sulfonylurea or TZD.

Continue to intensify every 3–6 months until the glycemic target is reached. While managing glycemic control, monitor all aspects of the disease and assess and manage microvascular and macrovascular complications of diabetes (see chapters 7 and 8).

SIGN recommends continuing a therapy if the target is achieved or the HbA1c decreases by 5.5 mmol/mol (0.5%) or more; therapy should be discontinued if ineffective.[1] The updated ADA/EASD consensus statement suggests stopping other drugs in preference to SGLT2 inhibitors or GLP-1RAs if at target.[2,3]

Intensification to injectables should be undertaken in primary care only by a health professional with training and experience in the initiation of these drugs. Otherwise the individual should be referred to a specialist team.

NICE currently recommends the use of GLP-1RAs in combination with metformin and a sulfonylurea if triple oral therapy is not effective, not tolerated or contraindicated *and*

- body mass index (BMI) is 35 kg/m² or higher (or black or Asian equivalent) *and* the person has specific psychological or other medical problems associated with obesity *or*
- BMI is under 35 kg/m² *and* insulin therapy would have significant occupational implications *or* weight loss would benefit other significant obesity-related comorbidities.[7]

NICE currently recommends that GLP-1RAs should be continued only if a reduction in HbA1c of at least 11 mmol/mol *and* a weight loss of at least 3% initial body weight is achieved at 6 months.[7] In real-world use, around 25% of individuals achieve both targets, with 50% achieving one of them.[9] Non-responders should have adherence checked and the drug should be stopped if there is no benefit. It is hoped that the NICE guideline update will bring it in line with the ADA/EASD consensus on glycemic management.

SIGN[1] recommends GLP-1RAs:

- as a third-line option if BMI is 30 kg/m² or higher (or equivalent for ethnic groups)
- in those with established ASCVD – a GLP-1RA with cardiovascular benefit should be used.

At the time of writing, liraglutide, semaglutide and dulaglutide have evidence for CVD benefit in those with established CVD.

When making the decision to initiate injectables, the ADA/EASD consensus recommends:[2,3]

- if HbA1c is above target despite dual or triple oral therapy and the person is not already on a GLP-1RA, consider a GLP-1RA prior to insulin
- if the HbA1c is above 86 mmol/mol (10%) or more than 23 mmol/mol (2%) above the person's agreed target, consider an injectable combination of GLP-1RA and basal insulin, or basal and prandial insulin
- consider insulin as first injectable only if
  - HbA1c is very high (>97 mmol/mol [11%])
  - there are symptoms or signs of catabolism suggesting insulin deficiency
  - type 1 diabetes is a possibility (if this is the case, ensure urgent specialist input at an early stage)
- if initiating a GLP-1RA, follow the directions on dosing and intensification
- if the person remains above the HbA1c target, add basal insulin or consider changing to a fixed-dose combination of insulin plus GLP-1RA – titrating against self-monitored blood glucose values
- if the person remains above their HbA1c target, add prandial insulin and titrate against self-monitored blood glucose values.

When initiating injectables, the ADA/EASD recommend continuing metformin and SGLT2 inhibitors. Stop the DPP-4 inhibitor if initiating a GLP-1RA. Stop a sulfonylurea or reduce the dose by 50% when basal insulin is initiated and consider stopping if prandial insulin or premixed insulin is initiated. Encourage awareness of the risk of diabetic ketoacidosis and highlight the importance of sick day guidance (see page 47) and risk of hypoglycemia (see chapter 4).

Glucose-lowering drugs

When choosing glucose-lowering therapies, consider the 'ominous octet' of defects contributing to hyperglycemia (Figure 5.4) and choose therapies that act on different defects.

The key information relating to glucose-lowering drug classes currently licensed in the UK is summarized in Table 5.2. Completed CVOTs that support the ADA/EASD consensus guideline recommendations are summarized on pages 117–18.

TABLE 5.2

Classes of glucose-lowering drug used in type 2 diabetes

	Hypo-glycemia	Weight change	Advantages	Disadvantages
Metformin (oral)	Low risk	Neutral	Inexpensive	Frequent GI symptoms Vitamin B12 deficiency Lactic acidosis Contraindicated with eGFR < 30; reduce dose if eGFR < 45
DPP-4 inhibitors (oral)	Low risk	Neutral	Well tolerated	Urticaria, angioedema (rare) Increased HF hospitalization (saxagliptin) Pancreatitis, bullous pemphigoid, arthralgia
• Alogliptin • Linagliptin • Saxagliptin • Sitagliptin • Vildagliptin				
SGLT2 inhibitors (oral)	Low risk	Loss	Reduce BP Effective at all stages if adequate eGFR CV, renal and HF benefits (canagliflozin, dapagliflozin, empagliflozin)	Mycotic genital infections/UTI Volume depletion/hypotension Transient decrease in eGFR Possible increased risk of fracture and amputation (canagliflozin, in the CANVAS Program only[10]) (Euglycemic) DKA (rare) Fournier's gangrene (rare) Care needed if renal impairment*
• Canagliflozin • Dapagliflozin • Empagliflozin • Ertugliflozin				

(CONTINUED)

TABLE 5.2 (CONTINUED)

Classes of glucose-lowering drug used in type 2 diabetes

		Hypo-glycemia	Weight change	Advantages	Disadvantages
Thiazolidine-diones (oral)	• Pioglitazone	Low risk	Gain	High durability No dose adjustment with decreasing eGFR Inexpensive Possible CV benefit (some groups)	Increased weight HF/edema Bone loss and fractures ? Increased bladder cancer ? Increased macular edema
Sulfonylureas (oral)	• Glibizide • Gliclazide • Glimepiride	Increased risk	Gain	Inexpensive Extensive experience CV neutral	Low durability Increased risk of hypoglycemia (major issue in CKD)
GLP-1RAs Exendin-4-based	• Exenatide • Exenatide once weekly • Lixisenatide	Low risk	Loss	No hypoglycemia as monotherapy	High cost Training to inject (all) GI side effects Pancreatitis and gall bladder disease (all; rare, uncertain)

			Advantages	Disadvantages
Human GLP-1-based • Dulaglutide • Liraglutide • Semaglutide	Low risk	Loss	No hypoglycemia as monotherapy CV benefits Possible renal benefits Can use to eGFR 15	As above Worsening retinopathy with rapid improvement in glycemic control in SUSTAIN 6 (semaglutide)
Human insulin	Increased risk	Gain	Highly effective	Training required Frequent dose adjustments
Analog insulin	Increased risk	Gain	More rapid onset of action	Lipohypertrophy and erratic absorption may occur

eGFR is expressed in mL/min/1.73 m^2.

*Do not initiate if eGFR <60; can continue to eGFR 45; the exception is canagliflozin, which is indicated at lower eGFR (see SmPC); only use lower-dose canagliflozin or empagliflozin if eGFR is <60; no dose adjustment is needed for dapagliflozin.

BP, blood pressure; CANVAS, Canagliflozin Cardiovascular Assessment Study; CKD, chronic kidney disease; CV, cardiovascular; CVOT, cardiovascular outcome trial; DKA, diabetic ketoacidosis; DPP-4, dipeptidyl peptidase-4; eGFR, estimated glomerular filtration rate; GI, gastrointestinal; GLP-1RA, glucagon-like peptide-1 receptor agonist; HF, heart failure; SGLT2, sodium–glucose cotransporter 2; UTI, urinary tract infection.

Selection of treatment should be based on effectiveness, safety, tolerability, individual circumstances, preferences, needs, indications and costs. If two drugs in the same class have the same efficacy, choose the option with the lowest acquisition cost.[7] Aim to become familiar with the benefits and potential adverse events and contraindications of one or more drugs from each class.

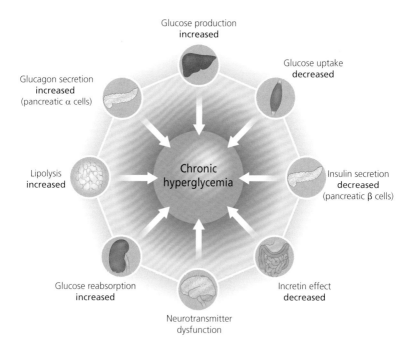

Figure 5.4 The ominous octet of organ and hormone dysfunctions that contribute to hyperglycemia in type 2 diabetes.

> **Practice point**
>
> Search for people with eGFR <45 mL/min/1.73 m² on full-dose metformin and people with eGFR <30 mL/min/1.73 m² who are still being prescribed the drug – adjust the dose or stop the drug.

Metformin is recommended in guidelines as first-line therapy. It decreases hepatic glucose production, increases glucose uptake by muscle and has other non-insulin-mediated mechanisms, including possible effects on gut hormones and the microbiome, that are still being clarified. Standard metformin is given twice or three times daily, while modified-release forms can be given once or twice daily. Reduce the dose by half when eGFR is below 45 mL/min/1.73 m² and stop when it reaches 30 mL/min/1.73 m². Metformin treatment is associated with lower vitamin B12 levels – check the B12 level if there is macrocytosis, anemia or neuropathy, and supplement if necessary. Metformin is available in combination with most other oral drugs, which can help reduce the pill burden. Metformin should be stopped temporarily if the person is undergoing a contrast study or is at risk of volume depletion (see sick day rules, page 47).

Contraindications include:

- current active or progressive liver disease (fatty liver is not a contraindication unless it is advanced)
- active alcohol abuse
- unstable or acute heart failure (not stable compensated heart failure)
- a history of lactic acidosis with metformin
- decreased tissue perfusion or hemodynamic instability (infection or other causes)
- lactic acidosis – the risk is low (9/100 000 person-years).

DPP-4 inhibitors act by inhibiting the DPP-4 enzyme involved in breaking down the natural GLP-1 that is produced in the intestine in response to oral glucose. These drugs therefore increase glucose-dependent insulin secretion and decrease glucagon secretion. If added to sulfonylurea or insulin therapy, there is a risk of hypoglycemia and the dose of the other drug should be reduced temporarily.

With the exception of linagliptin, the DPP-4 inhibitors are excreted by the kidney, so dose adjustment is needed to maintain therapeutic blood levels in individuals with renal impairment. There is no evidence of harm from failing to reduce the dose and these drugs maintain efficacy at lower eGFRs, unlike SGLT2 inhibitors.

When initiating a DPP-4 inhibitor (or GLP-1RA), advise the patient to seek medical advice if severe abdominal pain develops, as pancreatitis is a rare side effect. Check liver function in people treated with vildagliptin. Vildagliptin is dosed twice daily; all the others are dosed once daily.

SGLT2 inhibitors are once-daily oral agents that work by blocking glucose reabsorption in the kidney. They are therefore insulin independent and can be used at any stage of therapy, including, with caution, with insulin.[10-12] The glucose-lowering effectiveness depends on renal function – they are highly effective in individuals with normal renal function but only canagliflozin is currently licensed for use with an eGFR below 45 mL/min/1.73 m². All reduce weight and blood pressure as well as HbA1c. Empagliflozin and canagliflozin have benefits for major adverse cardiovascular events (MACE) in those with established ASCVD, and dapagliflozin, empagliflozin and canagliflozin reduce the risk of hospitalization for heart failure. Canagliflozin, dapagliflozin and empagliflozin have beneficial effects on indices of CKD,[13] such as slowing reduction of eGFR over time. Results announced from VERTIS CV with ertugliflozin suggest a CV safety profile consistent with other SGLT2 inhibitors, but VERTIS CV failed to demonstrate superiority over placebo in MACE or the chosen renal endpoint.[14]

SGLT2 inhibitors may be associated with an increased risk of dehydration and orthostatic hypotension, so caution should be exercised when used with diuretics, an angiotensin-converting enzyme (ACE) inhibitor/angiotensin II receptor blocker (ARB), or if the person has diarrhea/vomiting. SGLT2 inhibitors and ACE inhibitors/ARBs should be stopped temporarily if there is a risk of dehydration. It is not clear if the increased risk of lower limb amputations and fractures seen with canagliflozin in one trial,[10] but not subsequently,[15] are class effects; at the time of writing, a European Medicines Agency warning is in place.

Use with caution and contraindications. These circumstances are summarized in Table 5.3. Check the SmPCs (in, for example, the electronic Medicines Compendium at www.medicines.org.uk/emc) for individual drugs before prescribing.

TABLE 5.3

SGLT2 inhibitors

Should be used with caution (moderate risk) if:	Should not be used if:
• History of PAD or foot ulceration	• Previous lower limb amputation
• Frail/elderly*	• Existing foot ulcer
• Osteoporosis	• DKA or previous DKA
• History of fractures	• Eating disorder
• Ketogenic diet	• Excessive alcohol intake
• Cognitive impairment	• Rapid progression to insulin
• In combination with GLP-1RA	• LADA
• High HbA1c (>86 mmol/mol)	• eGFR <45 (do not initiate if eGFR <60); canagliflozin, 100 mg, can be initiated and continued at lower eGFR†
• BMI <25 kg/m²	
• On loop diuretics	• Acute illness
	• Pregnancy, planning pregnancy or breastfeeding
	• Recent major surgery

eGFR values are in mL/min/1.73 m².
*Empagliflozin is not recommended for people aged 85 or older because of limited clinical experience. BMI, body mass index; DKA, diabetic ketoacidosis; eGFR, estimated glomerular filtration rate; GLP-1RA, glucagon-like peptide-1 receptor agonist; HbA1c, glycosylated hemoglobin; LADA, latent autoimmune diabetes in adults; PAD, peripheral arterial disease; SGLT2, sodium–glucose cotransporter 2.
†See SmPC for details.
Adapted from Wilding et al. 2018[16] in line with SmPCs current at time of writing.

GLP-1RAs stimulate insulin secretion and decrease glucagon secretion in a glucose-dependent way, slow gastric emptying and increase satiety. Weight loss, glucose reduction, effects on fasting versus postprandial glucose and cardiovascular benefits vary between different drugs in the class.

Contraindications and special precautions. GLP-1RAs are contraindicated in: pregnant and breastfeeding women; children (liraglutide is licensed for children aged 10 years and over); and people with a history of pancreatitis or medullary thyroid cancer, or multiple endocrine neoplasia type 2 or New York Heart Association (NYHA) class IV heart failure.

GLP-1RAs should be prescribed with caution in people: for whom weight loss would cause concern (frail individuals, for example); or with untreated gallstones, inflammatory bowel disease or gastroparesis, renal or hepatic impairment, or retinopathy if co-treated with insulin. Recommendations for people with renal impairment vary – dulaglutide, semaglutide and liraglutide can be used down to eGFR 15 mL/min/1.73 m². Do not reduce the insulin dose rapidly when a GLP-1RA is co-administered.

Ensure women of childbearing age use adequate contraception (stop treatment before pregnancy – at least 2 and 3 months beforehand for semaglutide and prolonged-release exenatide, respectively).

Thiazolidinediones. Pioglitazone is the only drug in this class licensed in the UK. TZDs are effective glucose-lowering drugs, with durable effects, but are associated with fluid retention, increased heart failure, weight gain, fractures and possibly bladder cancer (avoid if undiagnosed hematuria or previous bladder cancer). Keeping the dose low may reduce the risks but is less effective for lowering glucose.

Contraindications. Pioglitazone is contraindicated in significant hepatic impairment and should not be started if alanine aminotransferase (ALT) is more than 2.5 times the upper limit of normal (ULN). The drug should be stopped if ALT is more than 3 times the ULN. Patients' liver function should be monitored.

Sulfonylureas lower glucose by stimulating insulin release from β cells in the pancreas, but this mechanism can have limited durability. Weight gain and hypoglycemia are the main side effects, with risk differing among the sulfonylureas available. Gliclazide is commonly used in the UK and has the lowest risk of hypoglycemia and potential for weight gain. Cardiovascular safety is uncertain, especially if

---

Practice point

Search electronic records for all those prescribed gliclazide. Review age, HbA1c and whether they appear to be undertaking self-monitoring of blood glucose. Review whether the sulfonylurea could be replaced by better-tolerated therapies.

PP

hypoglycemia occurs. The CAROLINA study demonstrated no increased cardiovascular risk of glimepiride compared with linagliptin (which had itself demonstrated cardiovascular non-inferiority compared with placebo).[17]

When initiating a sulfonylurea, ensure the individual knows how to undertake self-monitoring of blood glucose (SMBG), has a meter and test strips and knows when to test. Titrate the dose carefully against blood glucose to reduce hypoglycemia risk. Glipizide or glimepiride may be safest in those with CKD not on dialysis. In those with CVD, consider gliclazide if a sulfonylurea must be used; gliclazide is specific for pancreatic and not cardiac sulfonylurea receptors.

Hypoglycemia can occur at any HbA1c level as wide glucose fluctuations are common. The only way to identify hypoglycemia is through SMBG. Ask about hypoglycemia at every consultation and have a high index of suspicion in care home residents and the elderly, who may present atypically (e.g. with aggression or confusion). Hypoglycemia is more common in those with CVD, CKD, abusing alcohol, using aspirin concurrently or taking gemfibrozil or warfarin.

Reduce the sulfonylurea dose by half when adding any other therapy and consider whether to stop the sulfonylurea when initiating insulin.

Meglitinides. Repaglinide and nateglinide are short-acting prandial glucose regulators that are taken with food. They are more expensive than sulfonylureas, need to be taken three times daily and still cause significant hypoglycemia and weight gain.

Acarbose slows carbohydrate digestion and absorption from the gut, decreasing postprandial glucose. Gastrointestinal side effects occur in most users and limit therapy. Acarbose is not frequently prescribed in the UK because of adverse effects.

Insulin is an effective glucose-lowering treatment. However, the ADA/EASD consensus recommends that, unless the patient is very symptomatic, GLP-1RAs should be initiated in preference to insulin as they have been demonstrated to have similar efficacy with fewer side effects.[2,3] Weight gain and hypoglycemia are significant problems with insulin, with the latter often limiting therapy. Doses need to be titrated using SMBG results; significant insulin resistance can result in high doses being required, hence the development of U200 and U300 high-strength insulins. Human insulins are more cost effective than analog insulins but may cause more hypoglycemia, particularly nocturnal hypoglycemia.

Basal insulin given in the evening should be titrated against fasting blood glucose levels until fasting glucose is at the target. Prandial short-acting insulin may be needed with the largest meal, with additional prandial injections added if HbA1c remains above target. Consider premixed insulin with careful monitoring instead. **Do not initiate or intensify insulin unless you have been trained to do so and feel confident.**

The range of different insulin preparations, concentrations and delivery devices available means that errors in prescribing, dispensing and administration of insulin are a major concern, with potentially serious consequences that include death. The Medicines and Healthcare products Regulatory Agency (MHRA) has issued guidance that insulin should only be drawn up or administered using an insulin syringe and insulin should never be drawn up from an insulin pen device. NICE information on safer insulin prescribing highlights safety concerns, including the need for all insulins to be prescribed by brand name because of the availability of high-strength insulins and biosimilars.[18] Consider issuing an insulin passport that clearly documents the current insulin regimen. Drivers must notify the Driver & Vehicle Licensing Agency (DVLA) and understand their responsibilities for testing in relation to driving.

Health professionals who prescribe or administer insulin are encouraged to undertake safety training updates. 'Six steps to insulin safety' has been developed by the Primary Care Diabetes Society and comprises free e-learning modules and certification.[19]

Hypoglycemia. Everyone at risk of hypoglycemia (from insulin, sulfonylureas or meglitinides) should understand how to test for and treat hypoglycemia (see chapter 4).

Injection technique. Poor injection technique can result in bruising or infection of the skin and lipohypertrophy, which can result in erratic insulin absorption and glucose control. Best practice guidelines to support correct injection technique in diabetes care are available from Injection Technique Matters, an initiative run by TREND-UK.[20] Check injection sites, visually and by palpation, at every visit.

Key points – lowering blood glucose

- Guidance from the Scottish Intercollegiate Guidelines Network (SIGN) and American Diabetes Association (ADA)/European Association for the Study of Diabetes (EASD) should inform choice of drug therapy, as these incorporate the results from cardiovascular outcome trials. Guidance from the National Institute for Health and Care Excellence (NICE) is being updated (2019).
- Individualize and agree the glycemic targets.
- Tight early glycemic control reduces microvascular and macrovascular complications and provides a lasting 'legacy effect'; tight glycemic control late in the disease is more difficult to achieve and may cause adverse effects.
- Lifestyle modification and metformin are first-line interventions.
- Glucagon-like peptide-1 receptor agonists (GLP-1RAs) with cardiovascular disease benefits should be prioritized after metformin in those with atherosclerotic cardiovascular disease (ASCVD) or at high risk of ASCVD and sodium–glucose cotransporter 2 (SGLT2) inhibitors prioritized in those with chronic kidney disease or heart failure (particularly heart failure with reduced ejection fraction) with the other class added if the first is not tolerated or glycemic intensification is needed.
- When intensifying to injectables, use GLP-1RAs before insulin unless glucose is very high or the individual is very symptomatic.

References

1. Scottish Intercollegiate Guidelines Network. Pharmacological management of glycaemic control in people with type 2 diabetes: SIGN 154. Edinburgh: SIGN, 2017.

2. Davies M, D'Alessio D, Fradkin J et al. Management of hyperglycemia in type 2 diabetes, 2018. A consensus report by the American Diabetes Association (ADA) and the European Association for the Study of Diabetes (EASD). *Diabetes Care* 2018;41: 2669–701.

3. Buse JB, Wexler DJ, Tsapas A et al. 2019 update to: Management of hyperglycaemia in type 2 diabetes, 2018. A consensus report by the American Diabetes Association (ADA) and the European Association for the Study of Diabetes (EASD). *Diabetologia* 2020;63:221–8.

4. National Institute for Health and Care Excellence. Medicines optimisation priorities: key therapeutic topics. London: NICE. www.nice.org.uk/about/what-we-do/our-programmes/nice-advice/key-therapeutic-topics, last accessed 7 July 2020.

5. National Institute for Health and Care Excellence. Type 2 diabetes in adults: controlling your blood glucose by taking a second medicine – what are your options? Patient decision aid. www.nice.org.uk/guidance/ng28/resources/patient-decision-aid-1687717, last accessed 7 July 2020.

6. Holman RR, Paul SK, Bethel MA et al. 10-year follow-up of intensive glucose control in type 2 diabetes. *N Engl J Med* 2008;359:1577–89.

7. National Institute for Health and Care Excellence. Type 2 diabetes in adults: management: NG28. London: NICE, 2015.

8. Inzucchi SE, Bergenstal RM, Buse JB et al. Management of hyperglycemia in type 2 diabetes, 2015: a patient-centered approach: update to a position statement of the American Diabetes Association and the European Association for the Study of Diabetes. *Diabetes Care* 2015;38:140–9.

9. Hall GC, McMahon AD, Dain MP et al. Primary-care observational database study of the efficacy of GLP-1 receptor agonists and insulin in the UK. *Diabet Med* 2013;30:681–6.

10. Neal B, Perkovic V, Mahaffey KW et al. Canagliflozin and cardiovascular and renal events in type 2 diabetes. *N Engl J Med* 2017;377:644–57.

11. Zinman B, Wanner C, Lachin JM et al. Empagliflozin, cardiovascular outcomes and mortality in type 2 diabetes. *N Engl J Med* 2015;373:2117–28.

12. Wiviott SD, Raz I, Bonaca MP et al. Dapagliflozin and cardiovascular outcomes in type 2 diabetes. *N Engl J Med* 2019;380:347–57.

13. American Diabetes Association. Standards of medical care in diabetes—2020. *Diabetes Care* 2020;43(Suppl 1):S1–212.

14. Cannon CP, Pratley R, Dagogo-Jack S et al. Cardiovascular outcomes with ertugliflozin in type 2 diabetes. *N Engl J Med* 2020;383:1425–35.

15. Perkovic V, Jardine MJ, Neal B et al. Canagliflozin and renal outcomes in type 2 diabetes and nephropathy. *N Engl J Med* 2019;380:2295–306.

16. Wilding J, Fernando K, Milne N et al. SGLT2 inhibitors in type 2 diabetes management: key evidence and implications for clinical practice. *Diabetes Ther* 2018;9:1757–73.

17. Rosenstock J, Kahn SE, Johansen OE et al. Effect of linagliptin vs glimepiride on major adverse cardiovascular outcomes in patients with type 2 diabetes: the CAROLINA randomized clinical trial. *JAMA* 2019;322:1155–66.

18. National Institute for Health and Care Excellence. Safer insulin prescribing: key therapeutic topic. London: NICE, 2017, updated September 2019. www.nice.org.uk/advice/ktt20, last accessed 7 July 2020.

19. Diggle J. The six steps to insulin safety. Diabetes on the Net. www.diabetesonthenet.com/course/the-six-steps-to-insulin-safety/details, last accessed 7 July 2020. [Register free at www.diabetes onthenet.com/sso/register]

20. Hicks D, Adams D, Diggle J et al. Injection technique matters. Trend UK, 2017. https://trend-uk.org/injection-technique-matters, last accessed 7 July 2020. [Register free at https://trend-uk.org/resources]

6

Hypertension and dyslipidemia

Hypertension

Hypertension is twice as common in people with diabetes compared with those without; the combination of diabetes and hypertension greatly increases the risk of cardiovascular disease (CVD), including heart failure and stroke.

Diagnosis. The National Institute for Health and Care Excellence (NICE) issued updated guidance on hypertension in adults in 2019.[1] It recommends targets of below 140/90 mmHg for those under 80 years and below 150/90 mmHg for older individuals. When managing those with type 2 diabetes and chronic kidney disease (CKD), follow NICE clinical guideline 182, which recommends a blood pressure target of under 130/80 mmHg for this group.[2] Although the ACCORD BP (Action to Control Cardiovascular Risk in Diabetes – Blood Pressure) study confirmed further stroke reduction with systolic blood pressure down to 120 mmHg, there was no significant additional effect on cardiovascular risk; this has been taken into account in the updated NICE guidance on hypertension.[3] Recommendations for the diagnosis of hypertension in people with type 2 diabetes are shown in Table 6.1. Lower blood pressure targets are proposed in the European Society for Cardiology (ESC) guidelines on CVD prevention.[4] As both the NICE and ESC guidelines claim to be evidence based, the disparity has caused some confusion.

Management of blood pressure in people with diabetes is slightly different from management in the general population. An angiotensin-converting enzyme (ACE) inhibitor or angiotensin II receptor blocker (ARB) should be first-line therapy at all ages unless contraindicated (Figure 6.1); if the person has black-African or African-Caribbean family origin, favor an ARB over an ACE inhibitor.[1] Subsequent intensification of drug therapy is with the same drugs as in people without diabetes.

TABLE 6.1

Diagnosing hypertension

- Measure BP in both arms with appropriate cuff (bladder should be 80% of arm diameter)
- If BP difference between arms > 15 mmHg, recheck; if difference still > 15 mmHg, use arm with higher BP in future (CV risk may be increased)
- If clinic BP is 140/90 to 180/120 mmHg, use ambulatory BP or home readings to confirm hypertension (see NICE hypertension guideline)[1]
- If severe hypertension, BP ≥ 180/120 mmHg, and retinal hemorrhage, papilledema or life-threatening symptoms or possible pheochromocytoma, arrange same day review; otherwise, if end organ damage, treat immediately and arrange urgent specialist review
- Code hypertension; check height, weight, BMI, smoking status and history of CVD
- Agree BP target with consideration of risk of falls and hypotension
- Measure renal function (eGFR and ACR [urine]), lipids, thyroid function, liver function; use the results to calculate CV risk if appropriate (see chapter 8)
- Arrange ECG

ACR, albumin to creatinine ratio; BMI, body mass index; BP, blood pressure; CV(D), cardiovascular (disease); ECG, electrocardiogram; eGFR, estimated glomerular filtration rate.
Adapted from NICE 2019[1] (see guideline for further detail).

Lifestyle advice should cover weight reduction if overweight or obese, physical activity, not exceeding a weekly intake of 14 units of alcohol, dietary advice such as the DASH diet (see below), caffeine and salt reduction and smoking cessation.

The DASH diet is high in vegetables, fruit, wholegrains, low-fat dairy, fish, poultry, nuts and seeds, with sodium intake below 2300 mg and, ideally, below 1500 mg daily. There is evidence that blood pressure can be lowered with both salt restriction and the DASH diet, and the effects are additive.[5] Those with higher baseline systolic blood pressure (> 150 mmHg)

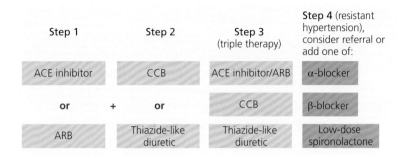

Step 1	Step 2	Step 3 (triple therapy)	Step 4 (resistant hypertension), consider referral or add one of:
ACE inhibitor	CCB	ACE inhibitor/ARB	α-blocker
or +	or	CCB	β-blocker
ARB	Thiazide-like diuretic	Thiazide-like diuretic	Low-dose spironolactone

Figure 6.1 Management of hypertension in people with type 2 diabetes. Check adherence at each stage before adding therapy. See NICE 2019[1] for further detail. ACE, angiotensin-converting enzyme; ARB, angiotensin II receptor blocker; CCB, calcium channel blocker.

get a greater blood pressure-lowering effect. Generally, reductions are similar to those achieved with a single blood pressure-lowering drug.

Drug therapy should be started with a once-daily generic ACE inhibitor. In people of African-Caribbean descent with diabetes, NICE now recommends starting with an ARB. For those with CKD and diabetes, follow the NICE CKD guideline. Women who may be at risk of pregnancy should start a calcium channel blocker.

Before initiating treatment, check the estimated glomerular filtration rate (eGFR) and serum potassium; repeat 1–2 weeks after initiation and after each dose increase. Do not initiate an ACE inhibitor/ARB if potassium is above 5 mmol/L and stop the ACE inhibitor/ARB at any time if potassium rises to 6mmol/L. A small drop in eGFR is common when an ACE inhibitor/ARB is initiated or increased. Do not modify the dose unless the eGFR declines by more than 25% or creatinine rises by more than 30%. If four therapies are required and spironolactone is used, monitor potassium carefully. Recent evidence suggests that taking blood pressure medication at night, rather than in the morning, is beneficial, but this is based on a single study.[6]

 Do not use an ACE inhibitor and ARB together.
ACE inhibitors and ARBs are teratogenic and must be stopped before conception or as soon as pregnancy is confirmed.

Refer for specialist advice if blood pressure is not well controlled with lifestyle changes and optimal doses of three or four drugs or if there are significant decreases in renal function with ACE inhibitor/ARB therapy.

Dyslipidemia

People with diabetes usually have elevated triglyceride, low protective high-density lipoprotein (HDL)-cholesterol and although low-density lipoprotein (LDL)-cholesterol and total cholesterol are usually normal, the LDL-cholesterol is small, dense and highly atherogenic. Consider the possibility of familial hypercholesterolemia; investigate and refer if necessary.

Pragmatic guidance on diagnosing and managing dyslipidemia is summarized in Table 6.2. NICE guideline 181 has further information; at the time of writing, it is being updated.[7]

TABLE 6.2

Diagnosing and managing dyslipidemia

Check

- Full non-fasted lipid profile, including: total cholesterol, LDL-cholesterol, HDL-cholesterol, non-HDL-cholesterol, triglyceride
- LFTs
- History of muscle pain (only check CK prior to statin therapy if muscle pain previously [see below])

Primary prevention

- If appropriate, use lipid profile to undertake CVD risk assessment
- Reinforce lifestyle advice
- NICE recommends offering statin if 10-year risk ≥10% and ≤84 years old
- Use atorvastatin, 20 mg daily*
- Offer statin without risk assessment if chronic kidney disease (eGFR < 60 mL/min/1.73 m² or albuminuria)

Secondary prevention

- Treat all without risk assessment
- Use atorvastatin, 80 mg daily

(CONTINUED)

TABLE 6.2 (CONTINUED)

Diagnosing and managing dyslipidemia

Statins

- Statins can be started provided:
  - ALT < × 3 ULN
  - CK is checked if previous muscle pain
    - If CK > × 5 ULN, repeat test within 7 days
    - If level remains > 5 × ULN, do not start statin
    - If elevated but < 5 × ULN, use low-dose statin
- Use the maximum tolerated dose
- If adverse effects occur, stop and restart once resolved; reduce dose within same statin intensity or change to lower-intensity statin
- Remind people that statin at any dose reduces CV risk
- Do not offer co-enzyme Q10 or vitamin D to improve statin adherence

In first 3 months after statin initiation

- Repeat LFTs
- Repeat lipid profile
  - Aim for 40% reduction in non-HDL-cholesterol or, as this can be difficult to ascertain, a non-HDL-cholesterol <2.5 mmol/L
  - Titrate statin if needed

Ongoing

- Repeat LFTs at 12 months (further testing beyond the initial 12-month review is no longer recommended unless clinically indicated)
- Annual review discussion on statin adherence (if targets are not met), can combine this with review for CVD and/or diabetes
  - Non-HDL-cholesterol measurement may help inform the discussion

*SIGN recommends atorvastatin, 10 mg daily, or simvastatin, 40 mg daily, for primary prevention in all those with type 2 diabetes aged >40 years regardless of lipid profile.[8] ALT, alanine aminotransferase; CK, creatine kinase; CV(D), cardiovascular (disease); eGFR, estimated glomerular filtration rate; HDL, high-density lipoprotein; LDL, low-density lipoprotein; LFT, liver function test; NICE, National Institute for Health and Care Excellence; SIGN, Scottish Intercollegiate Guidelines Network; ULN, upper limit of normal. Source: NICE 2014.[7]

TABLE 6.3

High- and medium-intensity statin regimens

High-intensity (decrease LDL-C ≥ 40%)	Medium-intensity (decrease LDL-C 30–40%)
• Atorvastatin 20–80 mg	• Atorvastatin 10 mg
• Rosuvastatin 10–40 mg	• Rosuvastatin 5 mg
• Simvastatin 80 mg	• Simvastatin 20–40 mg
	• Fluvastatin 80 mg

LDL-C, low-density lipoprotein cholesterol.
Source: NICE 2014.[7]

The recently published ESC guidelines on CVD prevention propose specific LDL-cholesterol and non-HDL-cholesterol targets for groups classified as moderate, high and very high risk.[4]

 Statins are teratogenic and must not be used in pregnancy. Advise women of the risk and stop 3 months before conception or immediately pregnancy is confirmed.

Risk assessment. QRisk 2 is the risk calculator specified in the NICE guideline, but QRisk 3 includes more risk factors; ASSIGN is used in Scotland – see chapter 8 for more information. Until NICE guideline 181 is updated, consider whether the 2019 ESC guideline on diabetes, prediabetes and CVD[4] provides more up-to-date guidance.

Statins are classified by how much they reduce LDL-cholesterol levels (Table 6.3), although they possibly also provide benefit by reducing inflammation levels.

The Medicines and Healthcare products Regulatory Agency (MHRA) warns there is an increased risk of myopathy with high-dose simvastatin (80 mg). As there are better tolerated alternatives, this medication is rarely used.

Communication. NICE provides a decision aid that can be used by and with individuals to help them decide whether to start a statin.[9]

Remind the individual not to drink grapefruit juice while taking simvastatin or atorvastatin. The drugs listed in Table 6.4 are metabolized by the liver enzyme cytochrome P450 3A4 (CYP3A4), which is involved in statin metabolism; if taken together, statin levels and the risk of myopathy and rhabdomyolysis increase. Follow the prescribing advice on screen at the point of prescribing.

Protease inhibitors, used for HIV infection, may increase the risk of developing CVD, but GPs are often not informed of an HIV diagnosis or treatment. Ask if the person is taking medication from any other prescriber or over-the-counter drugs and document the answer before initiating any drugs in primary care, but especially statins.

Other medications. NICE does not recommend the use of fibrates, nicotinic acid, bile acid sequestrants or omega-3 fatty acids, either alone or in combination with statins, for primary or secondary prevention of CVD.

TABLE 6.4

Drugs that potentially interact with statins metabolized by CYP3A4

Calcium antagonists	Anti-infectives	Others
• Verapamil	• Itraconazole	• Ciclosporin
• Diltiazem	• Ketoconazole	• Danazol
• Amlodipine	• Posaconazole	• Amiodarone
	• Erythromycin	• Ranolazine
	• Clarithromycin	• Grapefruit juice
	• Telithromycin	• Nefazodone
	• HIV protease inhibitors	• Gemfibrozil

CYP3A4, cytochrome P450 3A4.
Source: Catapano et al. 2016.[10]

Refer those who:

- are intolerant to three statins
- do not achieve agreed targets
- are not suitable for statins but have increased CVD risk
- have abnormal lipids:
  - total cholesterol is above 9 mmol/L or non-HDL-cholesterol is above 7.5 mmol/L
  - if triglyceride is above 20 mmol/L and this is not due to excess alcohol or poor glycemic control, refer urgently
  - if triglyceride is 10–20 mmol/L, repeat fasting test in 5–14 days; refer if level remains above 10 mmol/L
  - if triglyceride is 4.5–9.9 mmol/L, refer if non-HDL-cholesterol is above 7.5 mmol/L after management of risk factors.

Key points – hypertension and dyslipidemia

- Aim for blood pressure ≤ 140/90 mmHg unless there is chronic kidney disease, when the target should be ≤ 130/80 mmHg.
- An angiotensin-converting enzyme (ACE) inhibitor or angiotensin II receptor blocker (ARB) should be first-line therapy for hypertension unless contraindicated. Prioritize an ARB if the person is of black ethnic origin.
- Do not use an ACE inhibitor and ARB together.
- Blood pressure can be lowered with salt restriction and the DASH diet – adopting both gives the greatest effect.
- Use high-intensity statins for primary and secondary prevention in dyslipidemia.
- Women who may become pregnant should be informed that ACE inhibitors, ARBs and statins are teratogenic and advised to stop taking these drugs 3 months before trying to conceive.

References

1. National Institute for Health and Care Excellence. Hypertension in adults: diagnosis and management: NG136. London: NICE, 2019.

2. National Institute for Health and Care Excellence. Chronic kidney disease in adults: assessment and management: CG182. London: NICE, 2014, updated 2015.

3. The ACCORD Study Group. Effects of intensive blood-pressure control in type 2 diabetes mellitus. *N Engl J Med* 2010;362:1575–85.

4. Cosentino F, Grant P, Aboyans V et al. 2019 ESC Guidelines on diabetes, pre-diabetes, and cardiovascular diseases developed in collaboration with the EASD: The Task Force for diabetes, pre-diabetes, and cardiovascular diseases of the European Society of Cardiology (ESC) and the European Association for the Study of Diabetes. *Eur Heart J* 2020; 41:255–323.

5. Juraschek S, Miller E, Weaver C et al. Effects of sodium reduction and the DASH diet in relation to baseline blood pressure. *J Am Coll Cardiol* 2017;70:2841–8.

6. Hermida RC, Crespo JJ, Domínguez-Sardiña M et al. Bedtime hypertension treatment improves cardiovascular risk reduction: the Hygia Chronotherapy Trial. *Eur Heart J* 2019;ehz754.

7. National Institute for Health and Care Excellence. Cardiovascular disease: risk assessment and reduction, including lipid modification: CG181. London: NICE, 2014, updated 2016.

8. Scottish Intercollegiate Guidelines Network. Management of diabetes. Edinburgh: SIGN, 2010, updated 2017.

9. National Institute for Health and Care Excellence. Taking a statin to reduce the risk of coronary heart disease and stroke: patient decision aid. www.nice.org.uk/guidance/cg181/resources/cg181-lipid-modification-update-patient-decision-aid2, last accessed 7 July 2020.

10. Catapano AL, Graham I, De Backer G et al. 2016 ESC/EAS guidelines for the management of dyslipidaemias. *Eur Heart J* 2016;37:2999–3058.

Further reading and resources

Kirby M. At a glance factsheet: diagnosis and management of hypertension in adults: updated NICE guidance 2019. *Diabetes & Primary Care* 2019;21:121–2. www.diabetesonthenet.com/resources/details/glance-factsheet-diagnosis-and-management-hypertension-adults-updated-nice-guidance-2019, last accessed 7 July 2020.

Resources related to the DASH diet are available at www.dashdiet.org, last accessed 7 July 2020.

Low salt dietary advice is available at www.nhs.uk/live-well/eat-well/tips-for-a-lower-salt-diet/, last accessed 7 July 2020.

Diabetes UK has information prescriptions on blood pressure, lipids and glycemia that can be uploaded to clinical systems and personalized during the consultation. See www.diabetes.org.uk/professionals/resources/resources-to-improve-your-clinical-practice/information-prescriptions-qa, last accessed 7 July 2020.

7

Monitoring and microvascular complications

Monitoring

The nine key care processes described by the National Institute for Health and Care Excellence (NICE) and six additional care processes advocated by Diabetes UK are shown in Table 7.1. This checklist can be used to structure the consultation to ensure all results are reviewed and all processes are undertaken at least annually.

TABLE 7.1

Essential monitoring

Nine care processes (NICE)
- HbA1c (glycemic control)
- Blood pressure (cardiovascular risk)
- Cholesterol (cardiovascular risk)
- eGFR and creatinine (kidney function)
- Urine ACR (risk of kidney disease)
- Foot check (foot risk stratification)
- BMI (cardiovascular risk)
- Smoking history (cardiovascular risk)
- Digital retinal screening (early detection of eye disease)

Additional checks (Diabetes UK)
- Dietary advice
- Emotional and psychological support
- Help to stop smoking
- Structured education
- Flu immunization
- Sexual health (erectile dysfunction in men and pregnancy risk and planning in women)

ACR, albumin to creatinine ratio; BMI, body mass index; eGFR, estimated glomerular filtration rate; HbA1c, glycosylated hemoglobin; NICE, National Institute for Health and Care Excellence.

Achievement of these care processes was measured in the original NHS Quality and Outcome Framework (QoF) Diabetes domain and a limited data set informs QoF payments (England and Northern Ireland), with higher glycosylated hemoglobin (HbA1c) and blood pressure targets for those with frailty to prevent overtreatment. Data are collated by the National Diabetes Audit (NDA). The cholesterol target has been replaced by statin use for primary and secondary prevention. The most recent NDA data demonstrated that only 40% of people with type 2 diabetes were meeting the three 'old' targets for blood pressure, lipids and glucose required to optimize cardiovascular risk and just under 40% were meeting the 'new' treatment targets, including statin use. The importance of multifactorial intervention on complication and mortality rates is discussed in chapter 8.

Ensure the person with diabetes has input to every decision when possible. Monitoring and consultations at 3-monthly or 6-monthly intervals are appropriate until risk is optimized. For example, a blood pressure result higher than the agreed target would prompt monitoring and management by the healthcare assistant or practice nurse as per the practice protocol until control is achieved.

A more comprehensive checklist of medical evaluation at initial and annual visits was added to the American Diabetes Association (ADA) Standards of Medical Care in Diabetes 2020 (Table 7.2).[1]

Diabetic nephropathy/chronic kidney disease

Around 30% of people with diabetes have chronic kidney disease (CKD) compared with only 6.9% of those without diabetes.[2] The prevalence of end-stage renal disease is up to ten times higher in those with diabetes compared with those without.[3]

CKD greatly increases mortality, mainly from coronary heart disease. Excess mortality is low in those with diabetes without CKD, with 5% excess over 10 years. In the presence of CKD (albuminuria and eGFR <60 mL/min/1.73 m^2) there is 47% excess 10-year mortality.

Albuminuria is the earliest clinical feature of nephropathy and therefore it is important to diagnose it early. Once albuminuria occurs, the risk of cardiovascular disease (CVD) increases and continues to increase as renal function deteriorates.

Kidney function is assessed from eGFR and creatinine, while albuminuria/proteinuria reflects renal damage.

TABLE 7.2

ADA recommendations for diagnosis and monitoring

Assessing risk of diabetes complications*

- ASCVD and heart failure history
- ASCVD risk factors and 10-year ASCVD risk assessment
- Staging of CKD
- Hypoglycemia risk

Goal setting*

- Set HbA1c/blood glucose target
- If hypertension present, establish blood pressure target
- Diabetes self-management goals (e.g. monitoring frequency)

Therapeutic treatment plan*

- Lifestyle management
- Pharmacologic therapy (glucose lowering)
- Pharmacologic therapy (CVD risk factors and renal)
- Use of glucose monitoring and insulin delivery devices
- Referral to diabetes education and medical specialists (as needed)

Assessment of factors that increase risk of treatment-associated hypoglycemia

- Use of insulin or insulin secretagogues (i.e. sulfonylureas, meglitinides)
- Impaired kidney or hepatic function
- Longer duration of diabetes
- Frailty and older age
- Cognitive impairment
- Impaired counterregulatory response, hypoglycemia unawareness
- Physical or intellectual disability that may impair behavioral response to hypoglycemia
- Alcohol use
- Polypharmacy (especially ACE inhibitors, angiotensin II receptor blockers, non-selective β-blockers)

*Essential component of initial and all follow-up visits.
ACE, angiotensin-converting enzyme; ADA, American Diabetes Association; ASCVD, atherosclerotic cardiovascular disease; CKD, chronic kidney disease; CVD, cardiovascular disease; HbA1c, glycosylated hemoglobin.
Source: American Diabetes Association 2020.[1]

Diagnosis. Albuminuria, the earliest sign of diabetic kidney disease, is assessed from the albumin to creatinine ratio (ACR) measured in a first void urine sample. Diagnosing albuminuria (Figure 7.1) is important, as prompt management can reduce or reverse renal damage.

For a CKD diagnosis, eGFR assessment is needed. A non-fasting venous blood sample should be analyzed by the laboratory within 12 hours.[4] CKD can be diagnosed and coded if two eGFR measurements, made at least 90 days apart, are below 60 mL/min/1.73 m², with no intervening measurements above this threshold.[5] Finding an eGFR below 60 mL/min/1.73 m² for the first time should prompt a repeat eGFR within 2 weeks to exclude acute kidney injury (AKI). If the person is of African or African-Caribbean origin, a correction factor should be applied – multiply the eGFR by 1.159. Note that an individual's eGFR results may be influenced by factors such as dehydration, high muscle mass or consumption of a protein-rich meal.

Managing CKD. The key tasks are to:
- code and monitor CKD (see Figure 7.2)
- reduce the risk of AKI
- limit the rate of loss of kidney function
- optimize glycemic management
- review drugs and doses as eGFR deteriorates (see Figure 7.3)
- optimize cardiovascular risk reduction (see chapter 8).

Management is informed by the NICE clinical guideline on CKD (CG182) and subsequent updates and the updated ADA/European Association for the Study of Diabetes (EASD) consensus statement.[4,6,7]

Reducing the risk of AKI. People with diabetes and CKD are at increased risk of developing AKI. The factors that increase this risk are listed in Table 7.3.

If the individual is at risk of dehydration during intercurrent illness, specific medications should be stopped temporarily (see Table 4.5, page 49). Metformin may increase the risk of lactic acidosis, sulfonylureas increase the risk of hypoglycemia, and diuretics, sodium–glucose cotransporter 2 (SGLT2) inhibitors, angiotensin-converting enzyme (ACE) inhibitors, angiotensin II receptor blockers (ARBs) and non-steroidal anti-inflammatory drugs (NSAIDs) increase the risk of AKI. Patients can be reassured that these drugs are well tolerated at other times and help protect the kidneys. Ensure that drugs are restarted once eating and drinking has returned to the normal pattern. See NICE

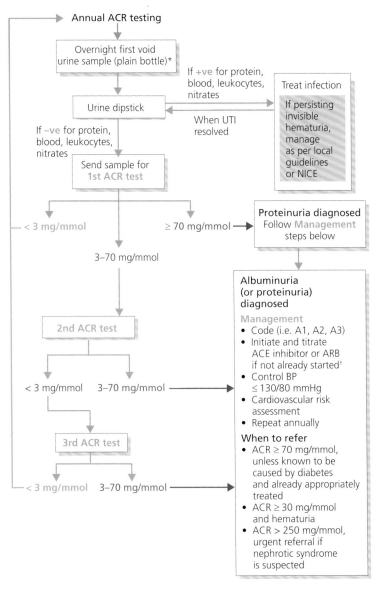

Figure 7.1 Diagnosing albuminuria. *If a first void sample is not available, request a random sample in clinic; if positive, request first void sample and send for testing. †Even if not required for hypertension management. +ve, positive; –ve, negative; ACE, angiotensin-converting enzyme; ACR, albumin to creatinine ratio; ARB, angiotensin II receptor blocker; BP, blood pressure; NICE, National Institute for Health and Care Excellence. UTI, urinary tract infection. Adapted with permission from Gadsby 2017.[8]

89

clinical guideline 169 for more information on the prevention, detection and management of AKI.[9]

Reducing the rate of loss of kidney function can be achieved by tight blood pressure control (≤ 130/80 mmHg) and treating with an ACE inhibitor or ARB. SGLT2 inhibitors and glucagon-like peptide-1 receptor agonists (GLP-1RAs) may also slow the rates of progression; canagliflozin is licensed for the treatment of CKD and further studies are awaited.[10]

 Do not use an ACE inhibitor and ARB together.

Optimizing glycemic management. The consensus of the ADA/EASD is that if CKD is present, intensification of glucose-lowering treatment after metformin should include an SGLT2 inhibitor with evidence of cardiovascular protection (see chapter 5).[6,7] There is some evidence from cardiovascular outcome trials (CVOTs) that SGLT2 inhibitors reduce albuminuria and progression of CKD, with greatest benefit in those with better preserved renal function (eGFR 45–60 mL/min/1.73 m^2).[11,12] Currently, with the exception of canagliflozin, SGLT2 inhibitors are not licensed in the UK for initiation if eGFR is below 60 mL/min/1.73 m^2. If already initiated, an SGLT2 inhibitor can be continued until eGFR is persistently below 45 mL/min/1.73 m^2, again with the exception of canagliflozin (see SmPC).

If SGLT2 inhibitors are not tolerated or are contraindicated, a GLP-1RA with evidence for reduction in CVD is recommended (e.g. liraglutide, semaglutide or dulaglutide, which reduced albuminuria in CVOTs[13-15]). Ongoing renal studies are needed to clarify benefits. This guidance has not yet been incorporated by NICE. Liraglutide, semaglutide and dulaglutide are currently licensed for use with an eGFR of 15 mL/min/1.73 m^2 or higher. Some SGLT2 inhibitors and GLP-1RAs also improve cardiovascular outcomes, which is important as people with CKD are at high risk of CVD.

Reviewing drugs and doses as eGFR deteriorates. At each eGFR measurement, check whether the drugs prescribed are still well tolerated (not just glucose-lowering therapy) and whether dose reductions are needed (see Figure 7.3). Metformin dose, for example, should be decreased at eGFR below 45 mL/min/1.73 m^2 and stopped if eGFR is below 30 mL/min/1.73 m^2.

eGFR category (mL/min/1.73 m²)	ACR category (mg/mmol)		
	A1, < 3 Normal to mildly increased	A2, 3–30 Moderately increased	A3, > 30 Severely increased
G1, ≥ 90 Normal and high	≤ 1	1	≥ 1
G2, 60–89 Mild reduction related to normal range for a young adult	≤ 1	1	≥ 1
G3a, 45–59 Mild–moderate reduction	1	1	2
G3b, 30–44 Moderate–severe reduction	≤ 2	2	≥ 2
G4, 15–29 Severe reduction	2	2	3
G5, < 15 Kidney failure	4	≥ 4	≥ 4

Figure 7.2 Recommended monitoring frequency per year according to chronic kidney disease classification by estimated glomerular filtration rate (eGFR) and albumin to creatinine ratio (ACR). Adapted from NICE 2014.[4]

TABLE 7.3

Risk factors for the development of acute kidney injury

- Previous AKI
- CKD G3+ (eGFR < 60; see Figure 7.2)
- Diabetes
- Age >65 years
- Liver disease
- Heart failure
- Sepsis
- Nephrotoxic drugs (e.g. NSAIDs)
- Hypovolemia/dehydration

AKI, acute kidney injury; CKD, chronic kidney disease; eGFR, estimated glomerular filtration rate (in mL/min/1.73 m²); NSAID, non-steroidal anti-inflammatory drug. Source: NICE 2013.[9]

Medication	CKD stage (mL/min/1.73 m²)				
	G1, G2 eGFR > 60	G3a eGFR 45–59	G3b eGFR 30–44	G4 eGFR 15–30	G5 eGFR < 15
Metformin			Reduce dose to 500 mg b.d.	**Avoid if eGFR < 30**	
Sulfonylureas	Gliclazide and glipizide preferred as metabolized in liver	Increased risk of hypoglycemia if eGFR < 60; consider reducing sulfonylurea dose			
Repaglinide					
Acarbose				**Avoid if eGFR < 25**	
Pioglitazone		Avoid if on dialysis			
Alogliptin		Reduce to 12.5 mg daily		Reduce to 6.25 mg daily	
Linagliptin					
Saxagliptin		Reduce to 2.5 mg daily; avoid if on dialysis			
Sitagliptin			Reduce to 50 mg daily	Reduce to 25 mg daily	
Vildagliptin		Reduce to 50 mg once a day if eGFR < 50			
Canagliflozin			Check SmPC		
Dapagliflozin Empagliflozin Ertugliflozin	Do not start if eGFR < 60	Stop if eGFR < 45			
Dulaglutide Liraglutide Semaglutide					
Exenatide b.d.		Increase dose from 5 µg to 10 µg conservatively			
Exenatide q.w.		**Not recommended if CrCl < 50 mL/min**			
Lixisenatide					
Insulin		Increased risk of hypoglycemia as kidney is main route of insulin clearance			

Figure 7.3 Dosing advice for glucose-lowering medication in people with diabetes and kidney disease. Consult the SmPCs before prescribing. For some medications, the threshold for stopping does not correlate with CKD stage. *Canagliflozin, 100 mg, or empagliflozin, 10 mg. b.d., two times a day; CKD, chronic kidney disease; CrCl, creatinine clearance; eGFR, estimated glomerular filtration rate (in mL/min/1.73 m²); q.w., once a week. Adapted with permission from GPnotebook 2018.[16]

Optimizing CVD risk reduction. People with CKD are at higher risk of CVD as soon as albuminuria occurs. It is therefore important to optimize blood pressure and glycemia, control lipids and encourage smoking cessation. See chapters 4 and 6 for discussion of these last two areas.

Referral for specialist care. People with advanced CKD have increased risk of anemia, fluid retention and heart failure, electrolyte imbalances and metabolic bone disease. Refer urgently if hematuria occurs at any time and for specialist assessment and management if renal problems are thought to be due to conditions other than diabetes (e.g. rapidly progressive albuminuria or in the absence of retinopathy or other microvascular complications). Further information is available in NICE clinical guideline 182.[4]
See also www.thinkkidneys.nhs.uk.

Diabetic retinopathy

Diabetic retinopathy is caused by damage to the small vessels in the retina which, in turn, causes ischemia, neovascularization (formation of new fragile blood vessels) and macular edema. Diabetic retinopathy remains one of the commonest causes of blindness in the working age population. Diabetic retinopathy usually coexists with other microvascular complications. In addition, glaucoma and cataracts occur earlier and more commonly in those with diabetes.

The main responsibilities and tasks of the primary care team include:
- explaining the risks to vision from diabetes and the importance of regular screening to minimize risk
- encouraging the individual to report any new eye signs or symptoms
- optimizing glycemic, blood pressure and lipid control to help reduce retinopathy
- referral to the retinopathy screening service at diagnosis
- actively managing non-attendance at retinopathy screening
- referral for immediate ophthalmologic assessment (qualified optometrist or acute eye clinic) if visual disturbance or eye symptoms
- referring for elective treatment if cataracts develop
- requesting preconception retinal screening for women planning pregnancy.

> **Practice point**
>
> When eGFR <60 mL/min/1.73 m², check that doses of glucose-lowering and other therapies have been appropriately adjusted.

Diagnosis. Historically, NICE has recommended annual retinal screening from diagnosis in those with type 2 diabetes. The Scottish Intercollegiate Guidelines Network (SIGN) recommends screening at diagnosis and then 2 yearly for those at low risk and annually for those with diabetic retinopathy. This pattern of screening will be adopted across the UK for those with no retinopathy in either eye.[17] It is particularly important that further appointments are arranged for those who do not attend. Non-attenders may be more likely to have uncontrolled risk factors,[18] so this group should also be supported and encouraged to attend the surgery for review.

Advice for patients. Encourage people to take all their glasses with them when attending for screening. Someone else should drive them to the appointment as their pupils will be dilated during screening and they should not drive until this wears off.

Screening classification. It is useful to understand the results of retinal screening letters and how people should be managed. Eye screening coding is shown in Table 7.4.

Retinal screening using digital photography provides 80% sensitivity and 95% specificity for the identification of retinal problems, but it is not 100% accurate. Visual problems that present in any individual with diabetes should be investigated, even if the person has not been diagnosed with retinopathy.

Risk factors. The main risk factors for diabetic retinopathy include duration of diabetes and poor glycemic control, so it is important to identify diabetes early and manage it optimally. In the UK Prospective Diabetes Study (UKPDS), tight glycemic control (glycosylated hemoglobin [HbA1c] 53 mmol/mol [7%] vs 63 mmol/mol [7.9%]) resulted in a 34% reduction in the development of diabetic retinopathy and a 17% reduction in progression among the newly diagnosed population recruited.[19]

The coexistence of hypertension, diabetic kidney disease, abnormal lipids and smoking increases risk, so these factors should be managed.

TABLE 7.4

NHS diabetic eye screening classification

Code	Findings	Management
R0 No retinopathy	None	None
R1 Background (non-proliferative)	• Capillary microaneurysms, hemorrhages, venous loop	• Inform GP • Continue screening 12-monthly
R2 Preproliferative	• Venous beading, reduplication • Intraretinal microvascular abnormality • Multiple 'blot hemorrhages' • Hard exudates • Cotton wool spots	• Refer to HES
R3A Proliferative (active)	• New vessels • Preretinal or vitreous hemorrhage	• Fast track to HES: sight-threatening emergency as risk of hemorrhage and retinal detachment
R3S Proliferative (stable)	• Stable retinopathy and evidence of peripheral retinal laser treatment • Stable preretinal fibrosis ± tractional detachment	• Monitor in digital surveillance clinic
M0 No maculopathy	• None	
M1 Diabetic maculopathy	• Retinal changes (exudate and thickening, microaneurysm or hemorrhage) within or close to macula	• Refer to HES or digital surveillance clinic • Can occur at any stage of diabetes

HES, hospital eye service.

Tight control of blood pressure in the UKPDS resulted in a 37% reduction in microvascular complications. It is uncertain whether the type of medication used to control blood pressure or lipids has an independent impact on retinopathy; until further studies are published, we should be guided by our ophthalmology colleagues, who will be following the evidence closely. Maintaining total cholesterol below 4.0 mmol/L, low-density lipoprotein (LDL)-cholesterol below 2 mmol/L and triglyceride below 2.3 mmol/L and initiating statins in those over 40 with retinopathy is recommended, although all targets should be individualized.[20]

In the LEADER (Liraglutide Effect and Action in Diabetes: Evaluation of Cardiovascular Outcome Results) and REWIND (Researching Cardiovascular Events with a Weekly Incretin in Diabetes) trials, there was a non-significant increase in progression of diabetic retinopathy in those with established retinopathy.[13,15] A 1.2% increase in absolute risk for retinopathy was demonstrated in a post hoc analysis of data from SUSTAIN 6 (Trial to Evaluate Cardiovascular and Other Long-term Outcomes with Semaglutide in Subjects with Type 2 Diabetes) in those treated with semaglutide who had pre-existing diabetic retinopathy and were treated with insulin.[21] This has been explained as relating to rapid decreases in glycemia in those with poor control and existing diabetic retinopathy at baseline.

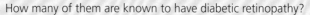

Practice point

How many people with type 2 diabetes in your practice have not attended retinal screening in the last 2 years?

How many of them are known to have diabetic retinopathy?

Prevention and management of retinopathy and maculopathy.
The following points summarize the approach.

- Tight glycemic control, ideally HbA1c below 53 mmol/mol (7%). (Vision may worsen in the first few weeks when glycemic control is tightened; in some cases this is due to osmotic effects on the lens rather than any impact on retinopathy. Vision should improve as glucose levels stabilize; the longer-term benefits are important.)

- Tight blood pressure control, below 130/80 mmHg if possible.
- Prompt assessment and referral of anyone with acute visual loss or new eye symptoms.
- Encourage those with advanced retinopathy who are already attending diabetic eye services to follow the advice they are given regarding driving and the types of exercise that are safe.

Consult the guidance from the Driver & Vehicle Licensing Agency (DVLA) on assessing fitness to drive in people with diabetes (see Further resources on page 110).

Intravitreal injections of potent steroids may be preferred for those with diabetic maculopathy, though this can result in increased cataract risk and glaucoma in up to 25% of people.

Intravitreal injections of anti-vascular endothelial growth factor (VEGF) agents are licensed for maculopathy; the PANORAMA study (Phase 3, Double-Masked, Randomized Study of the Efficacy and Safety of Intravitreal Aflibercept Injection in Patients with Moderately Severe to Severe Nonproliferative Diabetic Retinopathy) recently showed benefit in diabetic retinopathy without maculopathy.[22] Anti-VEGF agents carry a small risk of thromboembolic events and all intravitreal injections are associated with a very small risk of endophthalmitis, a serious infection within the eye.

Surgical vitrectomy is offered to some individuals with advanced retinopathy and hemorrhage.

Neuropathy

A variety of neuropathies can affect large or small nerves, producing a wide variety of symptoms.[23] At diagnosis of type 2 diabetes, 10–15% of individuals have neuropathy (as do a significant number with non-diabetic hyperglycemia); this rises to 50% by 10 years. Distal symmetrical polyneuropathy or autonomic neuropathy accounts for 75% of diabetic neuropathy. Up to 50% of sensory neuropathies are asymptomatic and undiagnosed, resulting in severe foot problems. The mechanisms for neuropathy remain unclear. See later in this chapter for more information on foot assessment and management.

The signs, symptoms and management of common types of diabetic neuropathy are summarized in Table 7.5.

TABLE 7.5

Common neuropathies in type 2 diabetes

Type	Signs and symptoms	Management
Distal symmetrical polyneuropathy	• Loss of thermal and pinprick sensation (small fibers) • Loss of protective sensation (10 g monofilament), balance, vibration sensation, ankle reflexes (large fibers)	• Tight early glycemic control to prevent or slow progression • Foot care according to classification of foot risk
Painful neuropathy	• Burning and pain	• Symptomatic treatment • Neuropathic pain medication for chronic painful neuropathy
Autonomic neuropathy	• Consider autonomic neuropathy if loss of glycemic awareness • Cardiac: asymptomatic, decreased heart rate variability, tachycardia (> 100 bpm), postural hypotension, silent MI • Gastrointestinal: any part of gut, gastroparesis, bloating* • Genitourinary: sexual dysfunction men and women, erectile dysfunction and retrograde ejaculation in men, full range of urinary symptoms • Gustatory sweating; lack of skin sweating	• Tight early glycemic control • Orthostatic hypotension: adequate salt intake; compression garments; care standing; encourage physical activity to prevent deconditioning • Gastroparesis: exclude other types of gastrointestinal problems first, small frequent meals, low-fiber low-fat meals, avoid drugs that slow gastric emptying; consider short-term erythromycin, domperidone or metoclopramide • Erectile dysfunction: manage testosterone deficiency if present; trial of PDE-5 inhibitor if no contraindications; refer if not effective

(CONTINUED)

TABLE 7.5 (CONTINUED)

Common neuropathies in type 2 diabetes

Type	Signs and symptoms	Management
Pressure palsies	• Carpal tunnel syndrome, or ulnar or distal sciatic nerve involvement may cause both sensory and motor symptoms	• Manage as for those without diabetes
Proximal motor neuropathy (amyotrophy)	• Progressive asymmetrical pain/weakness in hip, buttock and thigh	• Rare, refer for expert management
Mononeuropathy	• Diplopia if 3rd, 4th or 5th cranial nerves involved	• Refer for same-day specialist assessment

*Drug treatments, particularly metformin, remain the most common cause of gastrointestinal symptoms in those with diabetes.
bpm, beats per minute; MI, myocardial infarction; PDE-5, phosphodiesterase type-5.

Glycemic control. There is less evidence that tight glycemic control prevents neuropathy in type 2 diabetes than in type 1. There is no evidence of benefit once painful neuropathy develops. Rapid tightening of glycemic control may cause a temporary severe painful neuropathy.

Specialist referral. People with diabetic neuropathy other than distal symmetrical neuropathy or painful diabetic neuropathy will usually require referral for specialist care. This is particularly important for those with possible autonomic neuropathy.

Painful diabetic neuropathy occurs in 16–26% of people with diabetes and can significantly impact quality of life and sleep. It is more likely in those with a long duration of diabetes. Painful diabetic neuropathy can be difficult to manage, and it is important to encourage realistic expectations: 30–50% reduction in symptoms and learning to live with the pain using strategies taught by the pain clinic.

Painful diabetic neuropathy is a diagnosis of exclusion – always check blood tests for vitamin B12 and other causes, as these may be treatable. Management of neuropathic pain is shown in Table 7.6. Diabetic autonomic neuropathy may contribute to erectile dysfunction, which is covered in chapter 8.

TABLE 7.6

Management of painful diabetic neuropathy

- At each visit, take a detailed history, including a description of pain
- Undertake foot examination and monofilament testing
- Exclude and treat non-diabetic causes for neuropathy (e.g. vitamin B12 deficiency)
- Assess glycemic control (sudden tightening may trigger painful neuronitis)
- Initiate and titrate medication for neuropathic pain; if ineffective or intolerable side effects, switch therapies as recommended in NICE guideline[21]
- Offer initial treatment choice of:
  - amitriptyline (start at 10 mg at night and titrate; 75 mg daily is usual maximum)
  - duloxetine
  - gabapentin*
  - pregabalin*
- Undertake early review after treatment change to assess need for drug titration, adverse effects and efficacy
- Titrate to effective or maximum tolerated dose before trying another treatment; when withdrawing or switching, taper one treatment and introduce the new drug to avoid increasing pain
- Continue to assess and switch to second-, third- or fourth-line therapies as necessary
- Continue pain medication if it is working and undertake regular reviews
- Provide education about painful diabetic neuropathy

(CONTINUED)

TABLE 7.6 (CONTINUED)
Management of painful diabetic neuropathy

- At each review, check:
  - pain control
  - impact on lifestyle and activities
  - physical and psychological wellbeing
  - adverse effects of treatments
  - continued need for treatment
- Consider tramadol only as acute rescue medication
- Consider capsaicin cream for localized pain in those who wish to avoid or cannot tolerate oral treatments
- Do not use the following in non-specialist care – instead, refer:
  - *Cannabis sativa* extract
  - capsaicin patches
  - lacosamide, lamotrigine, levetiracetam, morphine, oxcarbazepine, topiramate, long-term tramadol or venlafaxine
- Consider referral to pain clinic if:
  - severe intractable pain not controlled by a trial of three neuropathic pain therapies
  - pain significantly limits lifestyle or daily activities including sleep
  - underlying health condition has deteriorated

*Pregabalin and gabapentin are now class C controlled substances, reflecting the abuse potential.
See NICE clinical guideline 173.[24]

Foot complications

Foot complications result from microvascular complications (neuropathy), macrovascular complications (peripheral arterial disease [PAD]) or a combination of both; they can be present at the time of type 2 diabetes diagnosis. Around 10% of people with diabetes will develop foot ulceration.[25] More than 135 diabetes-related amputations occur each week in England, with marked variation in the incidence of major amputations across the country.[26,27] Mortality rates are high following amputation, and amputation doubles the risk of further amputation. Ulceration and amputations can be prevented and reduced by good foot care; advise patients to make a same-day appointment immediately when foot problems arise. For an acute foot problem ('foot attack'), it is important to involve podiatry and foot protection teams and ensure prompt access to multidisciplinary foot specialist teams.

History and examination. Ask about previous foot problems including amputation and loss of sensation or burning, pain and numbness, cigarette smoking, known PAD, intermittent claudication, previous trauma to the foot and ankle or Charcot arthropathy, and presence of other microvascular complications.

Foot assessment and the management of foot risk and acute complications are summarized in Figure 7.4 and Tables 7.7 and 7.8.

Ensure all those who carry out foot screening have been trained and that you know your local pathway for referral and are assertive in getting people seen by a specialist team when required. Referral timings for acute foot conditions are summarized in Table 7.8.

Infection. If infection is suspected or being treated, refer to the multidisciplinary diabetes team.

Antibiotics. Follow local antimicrobial guidelines for choice and duration of antibiotic for infection. NICE has issued the following 'Do not do' guidance.[25]
- Do not offer antibiotics to prevent diabetic foot infections.
- Do not use tigecycline to treat diabetic foot problems unless other antibiotics are not suitable.
- Do not use antibiotics for more than 14 days for mild soft tissue infection.

Refer to the foot protection or multidisciplinary specialist foot team in line with local guidance.

Patients using SGLT2 inhibitors. The European Medicines Agency (EMA) has warned about a possible increased risk of lower limb amputations (mainly toes) with SGLT2 inhibitors.[28] Ensure people taking these drugs have a foot care examination prior to treatment and at least annually and are reminded of the importance of daily foot inspection and seeking advice if any discoloration, deformity, skin

TABLE 7.7

Foot assessment and management

Check the following

- Skin – dryness, cracking, discoloration, ulceration, temperature, lack of hair, nails, infection (check between toes)
  - If ulceration present, document site, ischemia, neuropathy, bacterial infection, area and depth (SINBAD) and arrange urgent referral
- Sensation – 10 g monofilament at five or ten sites (see Figure 7.4)
  - Test nearby site if callus at test points
  - If no response after three tests at any site, document loss of protective sensation (LOPS)
  - Change monofilament regularly and rest it between testing
- Circulation – dorsalis pedis and posterior tibial pulses; ankle–brachial index if appropriate
- Deformity – callus, corns, bunions, toe, foot or ankle deformities, prominent metatarsal heads
- Check for vision and gait problems and whether can reach/see feet
- Document and code findings in the patient's record
- Give advice and leaflets, including information on footwear and smoking cessation

Risk	Findings	Action
Low	• Normal sensation • Normal pulses • No deformity or skin changes	• Annual screening • Agreed self-management plan • Written/verbal information • Emergency contact numbers and prompt access if problems

(CONTINUED)

TABLE 7.7 (CONTINUED)

Foot assessment and management

Risk	Findings	Action
Moderate/increased risk	• One risk factor • No deformity	• 3-, 6- or 12-monthly foot check* • Individualized plan • Written/verbal information • Emergency contact numbers and prompt access if problems
High	• Previous ulceration • Previous amputation • Renal replacement therapy • Neuropathy and non-critical ischemia • Neuropathy and callus or deformity • Non-critical ischemia with callus or deformity	• Specialist foot check at frequency recommended by FPT • Individualized plan • Written/verbal information • Emergency contact numbers and prompt access if problems
Active	• Ulceration	• Rapid referral to multidisciplinary foot team
	• Critical ischemia • Gangrene • Spreading infection • Acute Charcot arthropathy • Unexplained hot, red, swollen foot ⊥ pain	• Hospital assessment/admission (see Table 7.8)
	• Painful peripheral neuropathy	• Individualized care with written/verbal information

NICE Quality Standard 5: all those with moderate- or high-risk feet must be referred to the foot protection team (FPT).
*As deemed appropriate by the podiatrist or FPT.
See NICE guideline NG19.[25]

TABLE 7.8

Referral timings for acute foot conditions

Immediate assessment by acute hospital team: limb- or life-threatening complications

- Ulceration with fever or any signs of sepsis
- Ulceration with limb ischemia
- Clinical concern that there is deep-seated soft tissue or bone infection
- Gangrene with or without ulceration

Refer to multidisciplinary foot care team within 1 working day*

- All other active diabetic foot problems

Immediate specialist assessment for consideration of immobilization

- Suspicion of Charcot arthropathy: redness, warmth, swelling, deformity (especially with intact skin), with or without pain

*Same-day discussion if presents on Friday.
Source: NICE guideline NG19.[25]

damage or pain occurs. Until the risk is clarified, do not use these medications in people with previous amputation or active ulceration and ensure detailed guidance is provided for those with high-risk feet. If people develop foot problems when taking SGLT2 inhibitors, stop the drug immediately and manage as described in this section.

Ulceration and amputation. Risk factors for ulceration and amputation are shown in Table 7.9.

Developments in care. The WIfI score is a risk score developed by the Society for Vascular Surgery. It looks at three major risk factors that impact clinical management and amputation risk in people with diabetic foot disease: wound, ischemia and foot infection.[29]

Other technologies, such as sensors and other detection systems, are in development and may help improve outcomes in diabetic foot disease in future.

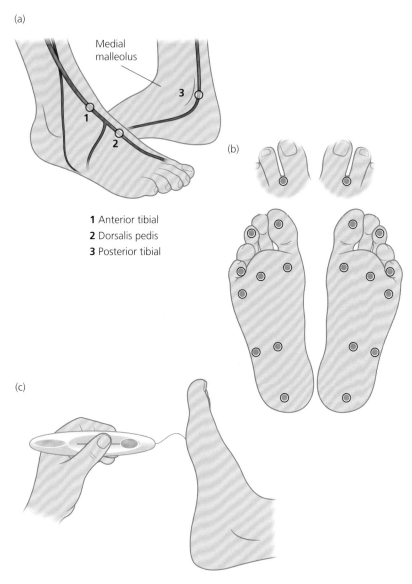

(a)

Medial malleolus

3

1

2

(b)

1 Anterior tibial
2 Dorsalis pedis
3 Posterior tibial

(c)

Figure 7.4 Foot assessment and risk assessment. (a) The major pulse points in the foot. (b) Sites for 10 g monofilament testing; five or ten sites are commonly used. (c) To test with a monofilament, place it at 90° to the skin; apply pressure to bend 1 cm; hold for 1–2 seconds and remove pressure; ask the patient to close their eyes and say 'yes' each time pressure is felt.

TABLE 7.9

Risk factors for ulceration and amputation

- Previous amputation
- Previous ulceration
- Loss of protective foot sensation (LOPS)
- Foot deformity
- Callus or corns
- Peripheral arterial disease
- Cigarette smoker
- Visual impairment (poor view of feet and hazards)
- End stage renal disease and dialysis

Key points – monitoring and microvascular complications

- The nine care processes recommended by the National Institute for Health and Care Excellence (NICE) should be undertaken at least annually for each individual.
- Tight glycemic control reduces the progression of microvascular complications but does not help painful diabetic neuropathy once established.
- Diagnose albuminuria and chronic kidney disease according to recommendations from NICE.
- Early diagnosis of albuminuria allows intervention to reverse albuminuria and slow progression.
- Risk for cardiovascular disease increases as soon as albuminuria develops and increases with deterioration in estimated glomerular filtration rate.
- Ensure people are referred for, and attend, retinopathy screening.
- Refer urgently for foot complications or potential Charcot arthropathy to reduce risk of amputation or long-term deformity.
- Have a high index of suspicion for autonomic neuropathy and ensure specialist input.

References

1. American Diabetes Association. 4. Comprehensive Medical Evaluation and Assessment of Comorbidities: Standards of Medical Care in Diabetes—2020. *Diabetes Care* 2020;43(Suppl 1): S37–47.

2. New JP, Middleton RJ, Klebe B et al. Assessing the prevalence, monitoring and management of chronic kidney disease in patients with diabetes compared with those without diabetes in general practice. *Diabet Med* 2007;24:364–69.

3. International Diabetes Federation. *IDF Diabetes Atlas*, 9th edn. Brussels: International Diabetes Federation, 2019. www.diabetesatlas.org, last accessed 3 July 2020.

4. National Institute for Health and Care Excellence. Chronic kidney disease in adults: assessment and management: CG182. London: NICE, 2014, updated 2015.

5. The Renal Association. The UK eCKD guide. 2017. https://renal.org/ information-resources/the-uk-eckd-guide, last accessed 7 July 2020.

6. Davies M, D'Alessio D, Fradkin J et al. Management of hyperglycemia in type 2 diabetes, 2018. A consensus report by the American Diabetes Association (ADA) and the European Association for the Study of Diabetes (EASD). *Diabetes Care* 2018;41: 2669–701.

7. Buse JB, Wexler DJ, Tsapas A et al. 2019 update to: Management of hyperglycaemia in type 2 diabetes, 2018. A consensus report by the American Diabetes Association (ADA) and the European Association for the Study of Diabetes (EASD). *Diabetologia* 2020;63:221–8.

8. Gadsby R. How to... diagnose, manage and monitor microalbuminuria. *Diabetes & Primary Care* 2017;19:13–31.

9. National Institute for Health and Care Excellence. Acute kidney injury: prevention, detection and management: CG169. London: NICE, 2013.

10. Sarafidis P, Ferro CJ, Morales E et al. SGLT-2 inhibitors and GLP-1 receptor agonists for nephroprotection and cardioprotection in patients with diabetes mellitus and chronic kidney disease. A consensus statement by the EURECA-m and the DIABESITY working groups of the ERA-EDTA. *Nephrol Dial Transplant* 2019;34: 208–30.

11. Zelniker T, Wiviott S, Raz I et al. SGLT2 inhibitors for primary and secondary prevention of cardiovascular and renal outcomes in type 2 diabetes: a systematic review and meta-analysis of cardiovascular outcome trials. *Lancet* 2019;393:31–9.

12. Perkovic V, Jardine M, Neal B et al. Canagliflozin and renal outcomes in type 2 diabetes and nephropathy. *N Engl J Med* 2019;380:2295–306.

13. Marso S, Daniels G, Brown-Frandsen K et al. Liraglutide and cardiovascular outcomes in type 2 diabetes. *N Engl J Med* 2016;375: 311–22.

14. Marso S, Bain S, Consoli A et al. Semaglutide and cardiovascular outcomes in patients with type 2 diabetes. *N Engl J Med* 2016;375:1834–44.

15. Gerstein H, Colhoun H, Dagenais G et al. Dulaglutide and renal outcomes in type 2 diabetes: an exploratory analysis of the REWIND randomised, placebo-controlled trial. *Lancet* 2019;394:131–8.

16. GPnotebook shortcut – medication in diabetes and kidney disease. *GPnotebook*, 2018. www.gpnotebook.co.uk/simplepage.cfm?ID=x201810177124437326, last accessed 8 July 2020.

17. Scanlon PH. The English National Screening Programme for diabetic retinopathy 2003–2016. *Acta Diabetol* 2017;54:515–25.

18. Leese GP, Boyle P, Feng Z et al. Screening uptake in a well-established diabetic retinopathy screening program: the role of geographical access and deprivation. *Diabetes Care* 2008;31:2131–5.

19. UK Prospective Diabetes Study Group. Tight blood pressure control and risk of macrovascular and microvascular complications in type 2 diabetes: UKPDS 38. *BMJ* 1998;317:703.

20. Broadbent D. Diabetic retinopathy: Fundamentals for primary care. *Diabetes & Primary Care* 2010;12:34–44.

21. Vilsbøll T, Bain SC, Leiter LA et al. Semaglutide, reduction in glycated haemoglobin and the risk of diabetic retinopathy. *Diabetes Obes Metab* 2018;20:889–97.

22. Anon. One-year results from positive phase 3 EYLEA trial in diabetic retinopathy presented at angiogenesis symposium. *PR Newswire* 2019. www.prnewswire.com/news-releases/one-year-results-from-positive-phase-3-eylea-trial-in-diabetic-retinopathy-presented-at-angiogenesis-symposium-300792822.html, last accessed 8 July 2020.

23. Pop-Busui R, Boulton A, Feldman E et al. Diabetic neuropathy: A position statement by the American Diabetic Association. *Diabetes Care* 2017;40:136–54.

24. National Institute for Health and Care Excellence. Neuropathic pain in adults: pharmacological management in non-specialist settings: CG173. London: NICE, 2013, updated 2018.

25. National Institute for Health and Care Excellence. Diabetic foot problems: prevention and management: NG19. London: NICE, 2015, updated 2016.

26. Diabetes UK. More than 135 diabetes amputations every week. 2015. www.diabetes.org.uk/about_us/news/more-than-135-diabetes-amputations-every-week, last accessed 7 July 2020.

27. Public Health England. Diabetes footcare profiles. https://fingertips.phe.org.uk/profile/diabetes-ft, last accessed 7 July 2020.

28. European Medicines Agency. SGLT2 inhibitors: information on potential risk of toe amputation to be included in prescribing information. 2017. www.ema.europa.eu/en/medicines/human/referrals/sglt2-inhibitors-previously-canagliflozin, last accessed 7 July 2020.

29. van Reijen NS, Ponchant K, Ubbink DT et al. Editor's choice – The prognostic value of the WIfI classification in patients with chronic limb threatening ischaemia: a systematic review and meta-analysis. *Eur J Vasc Endovasc Surg* 2019;58: 362–71.

Further resources

Driver & Vehicle Licensing Agency. Assessing fitness to drive: a guide for medical professionals. DVLA, 2016, updated 2019. www.gov.uk/government/publications/assessing-fitness-to-drive-a-guide-for-medical-professionals, last accessed 8 July 2020.

Selvarajah D, Kar D, Khunti K et al. Diabetic peripheral neuropathy: advances in diagnosis and strategies for screening and early intervention. *Lancet Diabetes Endocrinol* 2019;7:938–48.

People with type 2 diabetes have a two- to fourfold increased risk of cardiovascular disease (CVD) compared with those without diabetes. This can manifest as atherosclerotic CVD (ASCVD; acute coronary events and stroke) and/or peripheral arterial disease (PAD). Diagnosis of one of these conditions should always prompt careful history taking and/or assessment for the other conditions. Some complications may be due to a mixture of macrovascular and microvascular processes, such as diabetic foot disease, erectile dysfunction and heart failure due to diabetic cardiomyopathy.

Mortality and incidence of CVD are declining among those with diabetes, but the prevalence of type 2 diabetes continues to increase. Fatal outcomes are declining more slowly in those with diabetes than in those without. PAD and heart failure are now the most common initial presentations of CVD in people with type 2 diabetes.[1]

Prompt risk factor modification, including diet, physical activity and weight reduction, smoking cessation, prevention, diagnosis and management of hypertension, lipid modification and statin therapy, and antiplatelet therapy where appropriate, can reduce the risk of first and subsequent events and mortality.

CVD assessment and management
Key tasks to reduce CVD risk should be addressed (Table 8.1) unless an initial formal assessment of CVD risk is warranted (see below).

Assessment of CVD risk. Risk factors for CVD include:
• male sex
• smoking
• age over 50 years
• family history of early CVD
• certain ethnic family backgrounds (e.g. South Asian).

TABLE 8.1

Key tasks to reduce CVD risk in type 2 diabetes

- Reinforce lifestyle advice – diet, physical activity, weight reduction, smoking cessation
- Optimize blood pressure and lipids
- Optimize glycemic control – use specific drugs with cardiovascular benefit
- Offer platelet inhibition if appropriate

CVD, cardiovascular disease.

Individuals with risk factors and without previous CVD should have a formal assessment of risk; in England, this can be offered via NHS Health Checks. Potentially modifiable risk factors are listed in Table 8.2.

Risk calculators combine the impact of multiple risk factors to produce a 10-year or lifetime risk of CVD (see Further resources, page 129). Care and clinical judgment are needed when using risk calculators, as factors not captured may increase or decrease risk: for example, pretreatment with lipid- or blood-pressure-lowering agents. The 10-year risk score may underestimate risk in younger people and lifetime risk may be more useful.

Risk tools will underestimate the risk in those with:[2]
- HIV infection
- a serious mental health condition
- an autoimmune condition, such as systemic lupus erythematosus or rheumatoid arthritis
- dyslipidemia from medical treatment (e.g. caused by antipsychotic, corticosteroid or immunosuppressant therapies).

Where risk is calculated, different groups have made different recommendations for who is at high risk and needs treatment to modify risk. The National Institute for Health and Care Excellence (NICE) maintains those with a 10-year risk at or over 10% are high risk,[2] whereas the Scottish Intercollegiate Guidelines Network (SIGN) uses 20%.[3] Even at lower thresholds, lifestyle modification is appropriate. Code the 10-year or lifetime risk and the risk calculator used in the individual's electronic record.

TABLE 8.2
Potentially modifiable risk factors for CVD

- Diabetes
- CKD
- Hypertension
- Abnormal lipids
- Obesity
- Depression, anxiety and social isolation
- Lifestyle factors – low physical activity, smoking, poor diet, excessive alcohol intake

CKD, chronic kidney disease; CVD, cardiovascular disease.

Some people have risk factors that place them at sufficiently high cardiovascular risk for treatment without formal risk calculation. In this instance, although a risk calculation is not needed to make the treatment decision, the risk calculator can be used to demonstrate the benefits of lifestyle changes or medication. Individuals who do not need a risk calculation and should have treatment include those with:
- established CVD
- chronic kidney disease (CKD) with an estimated glomerular filtration rate (eGFR) below 60 mL/min/1.73 m² or albuminuria (albumin to creatinine ratio [ACR] ≥ 3 mg/mmol)
- familial hypercholesterolemia
- type 2 diabetes below age 40 years with albuminuria, retinopathy or neuropathy
- type 2 diabetes for 20 years or longer
- age 85 years or older.

Optimizing CVD reduction. To reduce CVD risk, multifactorial intervention is required (see Table 8.1, page 112). Each element is discussed below. The American Diabetes Association (ADA)/European Association for the Study of Diabetes (EASD) consensus statement also recommends prioritizing glucose-lowering drugs with cardiovascular benefit (see chapter 5).[4,5]

Although Steno-2 (Intensified Multifactorial Intervention in Patients With Type 2 Diabetes and Microalbuminuria) was a small study, it provided evidence to confirm that intensive multifactorial intervention, with small changes to multiple risk factors in those with type 2 diabetes and albuminuria, is beneficial in reducing cardiovascular events and mortality in the long term (Figure 8.1).[6,7] The benefit of a multifactorial approach has been confirmed in other studies.

It has been proposed that to reduce cardiovascular events, controlling blood pressure has more impact than controlling lipids

Participants
160 people with T2DM and persistent microalbuminuria randomized to intensive or normal treatment

Intensive treatment targets
- HbA1c < 48 mmol/mol (6.5%)
- Total cholesterol < 4.5 mmol/L
- Triglyceride < 1.7 mmol/L
- BP < 130/80 mmHg
- Low-dose aspirin
- ACEI or ARB (irrespective of BP; for microalbuminuria)

Study design
- Intensive treatment intervention versus normal treatment for 7.8 years
- Both groups received similar multifactorial treatment thereafter – followed for a further 5.5 years

Mortality rate
20% absolute risk reduction (50% vs 30%; $p = 0.02$)

Cardiovascular event rate
29% absolute risk reduction (60% vs 31%; $p < 0.001$); 59% relative risk reduction

Long-term effect
At 21.2 years of follow-up, those in the original intensive group had a median 7.9 years of additional survival

Figure 8.1 Steno-2 study design and results. ACEI; angiotensin-converting enzyme inhibitor; ARB, angiotensin II receptor blocker; BP, blood pressure; HbA1c, glycosylated hemoglobin; T2DM, type 2 diabetes mellitus.[6,7]

which, in turn, has more impact than glucose lowering.[8] Reducing blood pressure would be expected to have benefits within months and lipids within 1–2 years; the time to derive benefit from lowering blood glucose will depend on the drug class used.[6]

The UKPDS (UK Prospective Diabetes Study) supports the benefits of tight glycemic control **early after diagnosis** for reducing cardiovascular risk, microvascular complications and mortality. After glycemic control lapsed in the follow-up study, the group intensively treated initially had persistent reductions in microvascular and macrovascular complications, the so-called 'legacy effect'.[9] Although tight blood pressure control was, in the UKPDS, effective in reducing microvascular and macrovascular risks, there was no 'legacy effect' and benefits lapsed within a short period when tight blood pressure control was not maintained. It is less clear whether there are cardiovascular benefits or risks from tight glycemic control late in the disease in those with advanced type 2 diabetes and comorbidities; extremely tight control increased mortality in participants in ACCORD (Action to Control Cardiovascular Risk in Diabetes).[10]

Lifestyle interventions have been described in the self-management section (see chapter 4). Guidance on lifestyle for CVD prevention and management is the same as for type 2 diabetes management in general.

- Smoking cessation is a priority. Even if people gain weight with smoking cessation, this does not detract from the cardiovascular benefit, and this remains the same in people with or without type 2 diabetes.[11]
- Losing 5 kg has benefits for blood pressure, lipids and insulin resistance. A weight loss of 10–15 kg in DiRECT (Diabetes Remission Clinical Trial) resulted in many people achieving remission of type 2 diabetes.[12] People may choose to use less challenging methods than the 825 kcal liquid diet used in DiRECT and continue these longer term to achieve similar weight loss. Losing weight rapidly does not necessarily result in rapid weight regain, and early weight loss can predict overall weight loss.
- Both Diabetes UK dietary guidelines[13] and the ADA nutrition guidelines[14] include lifestyle advice for reducing cardiovascular risk in primary and secondary prevention.
- There is evidence of benefit for the Mediterranean diet for both the primary and secondary prevention of CVD events.

The Look AHEAD (Action for Health in Diabetes) study found that intensive lifestyle intervention produced weight loss, but it was stopped early because of lack of CVD benefit.[15] The study used a low-fat diet, higher in carbohydrates, which may not reduce cardiovascular risk. Nutrition guidance from Diabetes UK supports following a Mediterranean-style diet, with lower-carbohydrate options.[13]

Optimizing blood pressure. People with type 2 diabetes and hypertension are at increased risk of coronary heart disease (CHD), heart failure and stroke compared with the general population. The management of blood pressure is discussed further in chapter 6.

Optimizing lipids to reduce cardiovascular risk is discussed in chapter 6.

Optimizing glycemic control using drugs with specific cardiovascular benefit. The UKPDS demonstrated that intensive glycemic control with metformin from time of diagnosis of type 2 diabetes decreases risk of CVD in overweight and obese people,[16] though the impact on CVD may be less significant than previously identified. In a meta-analysis that included the UKPDS, intensive glycemic control was confirmed to be associated with a reduced rate of macrovascular events and all-cause mortality.[17] Metformin remains first-line therapy unless contraindicated or not tolerated in most type 2 diabetes guidelines.

In light of concerns that rosiglitazone might increase CVD risk in those with type 2 diabetes, the US Food and Drug Administration (FDA) and European Medicines Agency (EMA) have legislated that new glucose-lowering drugs must prove they do not increase CVD risk. This has resulted in large global cardiovascular outcome trials (CVOTs) with dipeptidyl peptidase-4 (DPP-4) inhibitors, glucagon-like peptide-1 receptor agonists (GLP-1 RAs) and sodium–glucose cotransporter 2 (SGLT2) inhibitors. In addition to confirming cardiovascular safety, CVOTs have found some newer drugs to be associated with a reduction in cardiovascular events (Tables 8.3 and 8.4). It is important to consider the baseline characteristics of the populations included in the studies, particularly the proportion who had established CVD as this group were obviously more at risk of future cardiovascular events and therefore may have benefited more. For example, in DECLARE-TIMI 58 with dapagliflozin, nearly 60% did not have established CVD at baseline (Table 8.3).[18] There was no significant reduction in major

TABLE 8.3

Cardiovascular outcome trials: SGLT2 inhibitors*

Study/drug/ follow-up	N (% with prior CVD)	HR (95% CI) for MACE	Comments
EMPA-REG OUTCOME Empagliflozin 3.1 years	7020 (100)	0.86 (0.74–0.99)	MACE result driven by reduced CV death
CANVAS Canagliflozin 2.4 years	10 142 (72.2)	0.86 (0.75–0.97)	
DECLARE-TIMI 58[†] Dapagliflozin 4.2 years	17 160 (40.6)	0.93 (0.84–1.03)	Reduction in co-primary endpoint of HHF/CV death

*Results from trials cannot be compared.
[†]This study had an additional primary endpoint of hospitalization for heart failure (HHF) and cardiovascular (CV) death, with hazard ratio (HR) 0.83 (95% confidence interval [CI] 0.73–0.95).
CVD, cardiovascular disease; MACE, major adverse cardiovascular events; SGLT2, sodium–glucose cotransporter 2.
Source: Giugliano et al. 2019.[19]

adverse cardiovascular events (MACE), but there was a significant reduction in the co-primary endpoint of cardiovascular death and hospitalization for heart failure (HHF). The results from CVOTs cannot be directly compared because of differences in study population and design.

At the time of writing, SGLT2 inhibitors and GLP-1RAs are licensed for glucose lowering and do not yet have a license for reduction of MACE or HHF. The updated ADA/EASD consensus statement (2019) suggests that GLP-1RAs can be considered in individuals without established ASCVD if they have specific high-risk factors.[4,5] Follow guideline recommendations – **do not extrapolate findings from CVOTs to groups other than those in the studies.**

TABLE 8.4

Cardiovascular outcome trials: GLP-1RAs*

Study/drug/ follow-up	N (% with prior CVD)	HR (95% CI) for MACE	Comments
ELIXA Lixisenatide 2.1 years	6068 (100)	1.02 (0.89–1.17)	
LEADER Liraglutide 3.8 years	9340 (81.3)	0.87 (0.78–0.97)	MACE result driven by reduced CV death
SUSTAIN 6 Semaglutide 3.1 years	3297 (83)	0.74 (0.58–0.95)	MACE result driven by reduced non-fatal stroke
EXSCEL Exenatide q.w. 3.2 years	14 752 (73.1)	0.91 (0.83–1.00)	
HARMONY OUTCOMES Albiglutide 1.6 years	9463 (100)	0.78 (0.68–0.90)	MACE result driven by reduced non-fatal/fatal MI
PIONEER 6 Oral semaglutide 15.9 months	3183 (84.7)	0.79 (0.57–1.11)	MACE result driven by decreased CV death
REWIND Dulaglutide 5.4 years	9901 (31.5)	0.88 (0.79–0.99)	MACE result driven by reduced non-fatal stroke
			(No heterogeneity between those with and without prior CVD)

*Results from trials cannot be compared.
CI, confidence interval; CV(D), cardiovascular (disease); GLP-1RA, glucagon-like peptide-1 receptor agonist; HR, hazard ratio; MACE, major adverse cardiovascular events; MI, myocardial infarction; q.w., once weekly.
Sources: Giugliano et al. 2019;[19] Cefalu et al. 2018;[20] Gerstein et al. 2019;[21] Husain et al. 2019;[22] Marso et al. 2016.[23]

NICE has not yet changed its treatment recommendations to bring them into line with the SIGN guideline and the updated ADA/EASD consensus statement, which specifically recommend prioritizing the use of GLP-1RAs for those for whom ASCVD predominates and SGLT2 inhibitors for those with CKD and heart failure. See chapter 6 for more details.

Antiplatelet therapy. Aspirin (acetylsalicylic acid [ASA]), 75 mg daily (or, if intolerant, clopidogrel, 75 mg daily) should be initiated and continued lifelong in those with a previous cardiovascular event. However, there has been uncertainty about the benefits of low-dose aspirin in primary prevention. In ASCEND (A Study of Cardiovascular Events in Diabetes), which involved 15 480 patients with diabetes but no CVD treated with 100 mg aspirin daily over 7.4 years, there was a significant 12% reduction in cardiovascular death, myocardial infarction, stroke and transient ischemic attack (TIA).[24] This was balanced by a relative risk (RR) of 1.29 for the primary safety endpoint of major bleeds, which were mainly gastrointestinal and extracranial. Two other large trials of aspirin, ARRIVE (A Randomized, Double-Blind, Placebo-Controlled, Multi-Center, Parallel Group Study to Assess the Efficacy and Safety of 100 mg Enteric-Coated Acetylsalicylic Acid in Patients at Moderate Risk of Cardiovascular Disease) for primary prevention in those without diabetes and ASPREE (Aspirin in Reducing Events in the Elderly) in the elderly (11% with diabetes), also found very small risk reductions balanced by significant increases in bleeds.[25,26]

In the UK, the guidance currently recommends aspirin only for secondary prevention, while the recommendation in the US is to discuss the risks and benefits for primary prevention, including bleeding risk. Dual antiplatelet therapy with aspirin and clopidogrel/ticagrelor/prasugrel is recommended for 1 year post cardiovascular event; drug selection depends on whether stenting occurs.

Stroke

Diabetes is an independent risk factor for stroke, with a fourfold higher stroke risk in those with diabetes. People with diabetes have a higher proportion of ischemic compared with hemorrhagic stroke; small lacunar infarcts due to small vessel disease are the most common type. Both cerebral small vessel disease and hypertension may contribute. Diabetes is associated with an increased risk of stroke recurrence, greater functional disability, longer admissions and increased mortality. There may also be a higher risk of stroke-related dementia.

Although hypertension alone increases risk of stroke moderately in those without diabetes, the risk increases with diabetes alone and diabetes with hypertension. Other risk factors include smoking and dyslipidemia. Hyperglycemia may occur early post stroke, probably reflecting the impact of stress hormones, and does not necessarily confirm type 2 diabetes.

In a subgroup of PROactive (PROspective pioglitAzone Clinical Trial In macroVascular Events), pioglitazone reduced both fatal and non-fatal strokes in those with type 2 diabetes and previous stroke. Liraglutide and semaglutide demonstrated reduced stroke rates in the LEADER (Liraglutide Effect and Action in Diabetes: Evaluation of Cardiovascular Outcome Results) trial and SUSTAIN 6 (Trial to Evaluate Cardiovascular and Other Long-term Outcomes With Semaglutide in Subjects With Type 2 Diabetes).[23,27] However, there was a non-significantly increased stroke risk with empagliflozin in EMPA-REG OUTCOME (Empagliflozin Cardiovascular Outcome Event Trial in Type 2 Diabetes Mellitus Patients),[28] although there were overall significant reductions in cardiovascular and all-cause mortality and MACE.

Heart failure

The Framingham study in 1974 identified a 2.4-fold increase in heart failure risk in men with diabetes and a fivefold increase in women.[29] Yet only in recent years has heart failure been considered an important cause of mortality and morbidity in people with diabetes. Heart failure occurs in those with previous ASCVD and hypertension – usually heart failure with reduced ejection fraction (HFrEF) – and also as diabetic cardiomyopathy, defined as heart failure without a recognized cause in a person with diabetes.

Type 2 diabetes and heart failure each independently increase the risk of the other, so those with heart failure – particularly those hospitalized for it – should be screened for type 2 diabetes. In diabetic cardiomyopathy, left ventricular dysfunction can be systolic or diastolic and pathological changes include fibrosis, advanced glycation endproduct deposition and damage to the myocardial capillaries. Autonomic neuropathy and lipid deposition in the myocardium may contribute. Heart failure occurs more commonly in those with diabetes and older age, longer duration of diabetes, insulin use, CKD and albuminuria, poor glycemic control and PAD.

Management. Supervised exercise training provided in a safe environment, such as cardiac rehabilitation facilities, improves symptoms in heart failure, as does intentional weight loss if obese. Heart failure with preserved ejection fraction (HFpEF) occurs in diabetes. For this group, unfortunately, only symptomatic treatment with diuretics is possible, as no currently available treatment has known benefits for mortality or morbidity.

In HFrEF, management is as for those without diabetes, namely diuretics, β-blockers, angiotensin-converting enzyme (ACE) inhibitors or angiotensin II receptor blockers (ARBs), eplerenone or spironolactone, ivabradine or the neprilysin inhibitor sacubitril combined with valsartan (in place of conventional ACE inhibitor or ARB, with specialist initiation). The benefits of ACE inhibitors and ARBs are the same with or without diabetes. There is no evidence for prognostic benefit of improved glycemic control in either type of heart failure. Pacemakers and implantable defibrillators may also be considered where appropriate.

In CVOTs, SGLT2 inhibitors significantly reduced HHF and cardiovascular-related mortality in those with type 2 diabetes, with a similar effect in those with and without ASCVD or baseline heart failure;[30] benefits occurred early after treatment started and they persisted.[28,31,32] In the glycemia management consensus statement of the ADA and EASD, SGLT2 inhibitors are the preferred treatment after metformin for those with heart failure provided the eGFR is within range (currently >60 mL/min/1.73 m² for initiation, with medication stopped if persistently <45 mL/min/1.73 m²).[4,5]

In DAPA-HF (Study to Evaluate the Effect of Dapagliflozin on the Incidence of Worsening Heart Failure or Cardiovascular Death in Patients With Chronic Heart Failure), people with and without type 2 diabetes with HFrEF (ejection fraction ≤ 40%) were randomized to dapagliflozin, 10 mg, or placebo for a median of 18.2 months.[33] The primary outcome, a composite of worsening heart failure (hospitalization or an urgent visit resulting in intravenous therapy) or cardiovascular death, occurred 26% less frequently in those treated with dapagliflozin, with a significant 30% relative risk reduction (RRR) in worsening heart failure and a significant 18% RRR for cardiovascular-related death.

Although some GLP-1RAs are associated with lower MACE, benefits occur over several months and are thought to represent an effect on ASCVD rather than on fluid load. There was no reduction in the rate of individuals hospitalized for heart failure with GLP-1RAs in CVOTs.

Thiazolidinediones should be avoided as they cause fluid retention and worsen heart failure. There may be an increased risk of lactic acidosis in those with heart failure treated with metformin. Saxagliptin is the only DPP-4 inhibitor shown to significantly increase the risk of HHF,[34] with a trend to increased risk with alogliptin.[35] Linagliptin and sitagliptin do not increase the risk of HHF.

Survival is poorer in those with diabetes and heart failure than in those without heart failure, with mortality as high as 30 per 100 patient years in older people (ten times the rate in those without heart failure). The 5-year survival is around 12.5%.

Erectile dysfunction

Erectile dysfunction, the inability to maintain a penile erection that allows sexual intercourse, occurs in up to 75% of men with type 2 diabetes;[36] management may be more challenging than in those without diabetes.

Men with type 2 diabetes should be asked about erectile dysfunction at least annually, and therapy discussed if necessary. The mechanisms contributing to erectile dysfunction include atherosclerosis and impaired endothelial relaxation, resulting in arterial stenosis and decreased blood flow into the penis, combined with inability to stop blood leaking out. In men with diabetes, a combination of neuropathy, vascular disease, endothelial dysfunction, hypogonadism and depression may contribute, as can therapies such as β-blockers, thiazide diuretics, antidepressants, statins and neuropathic pain medication.

Erectile dysfunction is an independent risk factor for coronary artery disease, as strong as hypertension and possibly stronger than albuminuria. All men with erectile dysfunction should have a full CVD assessment and aggressive management of risk factors. Other causes of sexual dysfunction occur in both men and women with diabetes, such as loss of sensation, lack of arousal and dryness, and enquiry should be made about sexual wellbeing at monitoring visits.

Management is as for those without diabetes. The impact of lifestyle changes other than smoking cessation are small. Phosphodiesterase type-5 (PDE-5) inhibitors are less effective in those with diabetes. Adding folic acid or arginine or using a PDE-5 inhibitor daily may increase efficacy.

Around 35% of men with type 2 diabetes have low testosterone levels;[36] a total testosterone level below 8 nmol/L occurs in around 15%. Testosterone replacement may improve quality of life, so consider referring those with very low testosterone levels.

Peripheral arterial disease

PAD is atherosclerosis in lower limb arteries and is usually diagnosed from an ankle–brachial index (ABI) below 0.9%. Of those with non-diabetic hyperglycemia, 20% already have an abnormal ABI compared with 7% in the general population; PAD affects one in three people over 50 with diabetes.[37] Cigarette smoking and diabetes are the most important risk factors, with increasing age, hypertension, dyslipidemia and CHD contributing. Among people with diabetes, risk is increased by longer diabetes duration, older age and presence of microvascular complications.[38]

Symptoms and signs include claudication, rest pain, ulceration and gangrene. The individual should be questioned about the presence and severity of symptoms of intermittent claudication and critical limb ischemia. Examine femoral, popliteal and foot pulses and measure ABI (Table 8.5). People with diabetes may present later, possibly because they are asymptomatic (because of peripheral neuropathy in some cases) or have atypical presentation, and have

TABLE 8.5

Measurement of ABI

- Patient resting and supine
- Record systolic blood pressure in both arms and posterior tibial, dorsalis pedis and peroneal arteries with suitable cuffs
- Use manual Doppler probe rather than automated system
- Document nature of Doppler signals in foot arteries
- Calculate ABI – divide highest ankle pressure by highest arm pressure for each leg

ABI, ankle–brachial index.

a poorer prognosis with increased amputation rates. It is not always possible to measure ABI accurately in people with diabetes because of calcification of the leg arteries. Do not exclude PAD in people with diabetes and a normal or raised ABI and do not use pulse oximetry for diagnosing PAD in people with diabetes.[37]

Management is similar to management in people without diabetes. NICE stresses the importance of providing information and ensuring people with PAD understand modifiable risk factors and self-management.[37] A subgroup analysis of EUCLID (Effects of Ticagrelor and Clopidogrel in Patients with Peripheral Artery Disease) outcomes in 5345 people with diabetes and PAD versus PAD alone showed a higher rate of MACE (cardiovascular mortality, non-fatal myocardial infarction or stroke), all-cause mortality and adverse limb events in those with diabetes and PAD. Each 1% increase in glycosylated hemoglobin increased MACE risk by 14%.[39]

People with PAD and diabetes deserve aggressive management of CVD risk factors (Table 8.6).

Consider prescribing naftidrofuryl oxalate if supervised exercise has not led to satisfactory improvement and the person chooses not to be referred for angioplasty or bypass surgery.[37] Review at 3–6 months and stop if no improvement.

TABLE 8.6

Management of risk factors in PAD and type 2 diabetes

- Support smoking cessation, as this reduces limb loss

- Offer long-term antithrombotic therapy with aspirin (ASA) or clopidogrel (but not dual antiplatelet therapy unless post MI) to all symptomatic individuals

- Offer the highest tolerated dose of a high-intensity statin

- Fenofibrate may reduce amputation risk (independently of lipid lowering)*

- If affected by intermittent claudication, offer a supervised exercise programme, ideally 2 hours weekly for 3 months; encourage people to exercise to the point of maximal pain

*Rajamani et al. 2009.[40]
ASA, acetylsalicylic acid; MI, myocardial infarction;
PAD, peripheral arterial disease.

 SGLT2 inhibitors may increase the risk of amputation in people with type 2 diabetes and PAD. Use with extreme caution or avoid using in PAD until further information is available, particularly if the person has had a previous amputation.

Imaging and revascularization criteria are as for those without diabetes, but there may be more distal disease, making surgery more difficult.

Careful foot care and prompt management of ulceration can reduce amputation risk. Ensure everyone with critical limb ischemia is admitted or immediately assessed by a vascular surgeon.

Critical limb ischemic pain. Offer appropriate analgesia to people with critical limb ischemic pain.

Key points – macrovascular complications

- People with diabetes have a two- to fourfold increased risk of cardiovascular disease (CVD) compared with those without diabetes. This may present as atherosclerotic CVD (acute coronary events and stroke), erectile dysfunction and/or peripheral arterial disease (PAD).
- Undertake a CVD risk assessment (unless at very high risk, when all should be treated), optimize lifestyle, manage glycemia, blood pressure and lipids, and initiate antiplatelet therapy if appropriate.
- If established CVD or specific high-risk factors for CVD, consider a glucagon-like peptide-1 receptor agonist (GLP-1RA) with evidence of cardiovascular benefits as second-line treatment after metformin.
- Erectile dysfunction is more difficult to treat in those with type 2 diabetes. Use phosphodiesterase type-5 (PDE-5) inhibitors. Refer men with very low testosterone as testosterone replacement therapy may be warranted.
- The diagnosis of PAD is confirmed with ankle–brachial index below 0.9%, but note that calcification of leg arteries in diabetes may give a falsely high result. Smoking cessation, single antiplatelet agent and supervised exercise programme are the mainstays of treatment.
- Currently, SGLT2 inhibitors should be avoided or used with extreme caution in those with PAD, previous amputation or active ulceration because of a possible increase in risk of amputations. Further guidance is awaited.

References

1. Shah AD, Langenberg C, Rapsomanıkı E et al. Type 2 diabetes and incidence of cardiovascular diseases: a cohort study in 1.9 million people. *Lancet Diabetes Endocrinol* 2015;3:105–13.

2. National Institute for Health and Care Excellence. Cardiovascular disease: risk assessment and reduction, including lipid modification (CG181). London: NICE, 2014, updated 2016.

3. Scottish Intercollegiate Guidelines Network. Risk estimation and the prevention of cardiovascular disease: SIGN 149. Edinburgh: SIGN, 2017.

4. Davies M, D'Alessio D, Fradkin J et al. Management of hyperglycemia in type 2 diabetes, 2018. A consensus report by the American Diabetes Association (ADA) and the European Association for the Study of Diabetes (EASD). *Diabetes Care* 2018; 41:2669–701.

5. Buse JB, Wexler DJ, Tsapas A et al. 2019 update to: Management of hyperglycaemia in type 2 diabetes, 2018. A consensus report by the American Diabetes Association (ADA) and the European Association for the Study of Diabetes (EASD). *Diabetologia* 2020;63:221–8.

6. Gaede P, Lund-Andersen H, Parving HH et al. Effect of a multifactorial intervention on mortality in type 2 diabetes. *N Engl J Med* 2008;358:580–91.

7. Gaede P, Oellgaard J, Carstensen B et al. Years of life gained by multifactorial intervention in patients with type 2 diabetes mellitus and microalbuminuria: 21 years follow up on the Steno-2 randomised trial. *Diabetologia* 2016;59:2298–307.

8. Yudkin JS, Richter B, Gale EA. Intensified glucose lowering in type 2 diabetes: time for a reappraisal. *Diabetologia* 2010;53:2079–85.

9. Holman RR, Paul SK, Bethel MA et al. 10-year follow-up of intensive glucose control in type 2 diabetes. *N Engl J Med* 2008;359:1577–89.

10. ACCORD Study Group, Gerstein HC, Miller ME et al. Long-term effects of intensive glucose lowering on cardiovascular outcomes. *N Engl J Med* 2011;364:818–28.

11. Clair C, Rigotti NA, Porneala B et al. Association of smoking cessation and weight change with cardiovascular disease among adults with and without diabetes. *JAMA* 2013;309:1014–21.

12. Lean MEJ, Leslie WS, Barnes AC et al. Primary care-led weight management for remission of type 2 diabetes (DiRECT): an open-label, cluster-randomised trial. *Lancet* 2018;391:541–51.

13. Diabetes UK. Evidence-based nutrition guidelines for the prevention and management of diabetes. 2018. www.diabetes.org.uk/professionals/position-statements-reports/food-nutrition-lifestyle/evidence-based-nutrition-guidelines-for-the-prevention-and-management-of-diabetes, last accessed 8 July 2020.

14. Evert AB, Dennison M, Gardner CD et al. Nutrition therapy for adults with diabetes or prediabetes: a consensus report. *Diabetes Care* 2019;42:731–54.

15. Dutton GR, Lewis CE. The Look AHEAD trial: implications for lifestyle intervention in type 2 diabetes mellitus. *Prog Cardiovasc Dis* 2015;58:69–75.

16. Stratton IM, Adler AI, Neil HAW et al. Association of glycaemia with macrovascular and microvascular complications of type 2 diabetes (UKPDS 35): prospective observational study. *BMJ* 2000;321:405–12.

17. Ray KK, Seshasai SR, Wijesuriya S et al. Effect of intensive control of glucose on cardiovascular outcomes and death in patients with diabetes mellitus: a meta-analysis of randomised controlled trials. *Lancet* 2009;373:1765–72.

18. Wiviott SD, Raz I, Bonaca MP et al. Dapagliflozin and cardiovascular outcomes in type 2 diabetes. *N Engl J Med* 2018;380: 347–57.

19. Giugliano D, Maiorino MI, Bellastella G et al. Glycemic control, preexisting cardiovascular disease, and risk of major cardiovascular events in patients with type 2 diabetes mellitus: systematic review with meta-analysis of cardiovascular outcome trials and intensive glucose control trials. *J Am Heart Assoc* 2019;8:e012356.

20. Cefalu WT, Kaul S, Hertzel C et al. Cardiovascular outcomes trials in type 2 diabetes: where do we go from here? Reflections from a Diabetes Care Editors' Expert Forum. *Diabetes Care* 2018;41:14–31.

21. Gerstein HC, Colhoun HM, Dagenais GR et al. Dulaglutide and cardiovascular outcomes in type 2 diabetes (REWIND): a double-blind, randomised placebo-controlled trial. *Lancet* 2019;394:121–30.

22. Husain M, Birkenfeld AL, Donsmark M et al. Oral semaglutide and cardiovascular outcomes in patients with type 2 diabetes. *N Engl J Med* 2019;381:841–51.

23. Marso SP, Daniels GH, Brown-Frandsen K et al. Liraglutide and cardiovascular outcomes in type 2 diabetes. *N Engl J Med* 2016;375:311–22.

24. ASCEND Study Collaborative Group, Bowman L, Mafham M et al. Effects of aspirin for primary prevention in persons with diabetes mellitus. *New Engl J Med* 2018;379:1529–39.

25. Gaziano JM, Brotons C, Coppolecchia R et al. Use of aspirin to reduce risk of initial vascular events in patients at moderate risk of cardiovascular disease (ARRIVE): a randomised, double-blind, placebo-controlled trial. *Lancet* 2018;392:1036–46.

26. McNeil JJ, Wolfe R, Woods RL et al. Effect of aspirin on cardiovascular events and bleeding in the healthy elderly. *N Engl J Med* 2018;379:1509–18.

27. Marso SP, Bain SC, Consoli A et al. Semaglutide and cardiovascular outcomes in patients with type 2 diabetes. *N Engl J Med* 2016;375:1834–44.

28. Zinman B, Wanner C, Lachin JM et al. Empagliflozin, cardiovascular outcomes and mortality in type 2 diabetes. *N Engl J Med* 2015;373:2117–28.

29. Kannel WB, Hjortland M, Castelli WP. Role of diabetes in congestive heart failure: the Framingham study. *Am J Cardiol* 1974;34:29–34.

30. Zelniker TA, Wiviott SD, Raz I et al. SGLT2 inibitors for primary and secondary prevention of cardiovascular and renal outcomes in type 2 diabetes: a systematic review and meta-analysis of cardiovascular outcome trials. *Lancet* 2019;393:31–9.

31. Neal B, Perkovic V, Mahaffey KW et al. Canagliflozin and cardiovascular and renal events in type 2 diabetes. *N Engl J Med* 2017;377:644–57.

32. Wiviott SD, Raz I, Bonaca MP et al. Dapagliflozin and cardiovascular outcomes in type 2 diabetes. *N Engl J Med* 2019;380: 347–57.

33. McMurray JVJ, Solomon SD, Inzucch SE et al. Dapagliflozin in patients with heart failure and reduced ejection fraction. *N Engl J Med* 2019;381:1995–2008.

34. Scirica B, Bhatt D, Braunwald E et al. Saxagliptin and cardiovascular outcomes in patients with type 2 diabetes mellitus. *N Engl J Med* 2013;369:1317–26.

35. White WB, Cannon CP, Heller SR et al. Alogliptin after acute coronary syndrome in patients with type 2 diabetes. *N Engl J Med* 2013;369:1327–35.

36. Hackett GI. Erectile dysfunction, diabetes and cardiovascular risk. *Br J Diabetes* 2016;16:52–7.

37. National Institute for Health and Care Excellence. Peripheral arterial disease: diagnosis and management: CG147. London: NICE, 2012, updated 2018.

38. Nativel M, Potier L, Alexandre L et al. Lower extremity arterial disease in patients with diabetes: a contemporary narrative review. *Cardiovasc Diabetol* 2018;17:138.

39. Low Wang CC, Blomster JI, Heizer G et al. Cardiovascular and limb outcomes in patients with diabetes and peripheral artery disease: the EUCLID trial. *J Am Coll Cardiol* 2018;72:3274–84.

40. Rajamani K, Colman PG, Li LP et al. Effect of fenofibrate on amputation events in people with type 2 diabetes mellitus (FIELD study): a prespecified analysis of a randomised controlled trial. *Lancet* 2009;373:1780–8.

Further resources: CVD risk calculators

QRISK®-lifetime cardiovascular risk calculator. Available at: https://qrisk.org/lifetime/

QRISK®3-2018 risk calculator. Available at: https://qrisk.org/three/

Joint British Societies for the Prevention of Cardiovascular Disease. JBS3 risk calculator. Available at: www.jbs3risk.com/pages/risk_calculator.htm

ASSIGN risk calculator, developed by Dundee University. Available at: www.assign-score.com/estimate-the-risk/

Children

Type 2 diabetes is increasingly diagnosed in children and young people; the predisposing factors include female sex, family history, ethnicity and obesity. Surveillance data from 2015/16 put the incidence in children under 17 years of age in the UK at 0.72/100 000.[1] Although children of all ethnicities were affected, incidence was highest among Asian and black/African/Caribbean/black British children, with more girls affected (67%) than boys. Most children – 81% – had a family history of type 2 diabetes (70% with a first-degree relative) and 96% were overweight or obese.[1]

Type 2 diabetes runs a more aggressive course in children than in adults, with the overall risk of complications being higher than for adults with type 2 diabetes or children with type 1 diabetes.[2,3]

Presentation. In the 2015/16 survey, just over one-third of children were asymptomatic, being diagnosed subsequent to an incidental glucose result or assessment for obesity-related comorbidities.[1] Children and young people with possible type 2 diabetes are often identified in community clinics.[4]

Around half of the children identified in 2015/16 experienced the classic symptoms – polyuria, nocturia, polydipsia and/or weight loss – and half had evidence of ketonuria.[1] Just under one-fifth had recurrent infections, with genital/perineal infections being the most common. Cellulitis, skin abscess and urinary tract infection were also present at diagnosis in some children.[1] The comorbidities evident at diagnosis are shown in Table 9.1.

Diagnosis. The 2015 guidance from the National Institute for Health and Care Excellence (NICE) on diabetes in children and young people[5] – the first to look at type 2 diabetes in this age group – recommends that type 1 diabetes should be assumed unless there are

TABLE 9.1

Comorbidities in UK children at diagnosis with type 2 diabetes

- Non-alcoholic fatty liver disease, 37%
- Hypertension, 21%
- Dyslipidemia, 9%
- Renal disease, 3%
- Psychological comorbidities, 2%

Source: Candler et al. 2018.[1]

strong indicators of type 2 diabetes; these include:
- family history
- obesity
- black or Asian ethnic background
- no requirement for insulin, or requirement is < 0.5 U/kg/day after partial remission phase
- evidence of insulin resistance (the presence of acanthosis nigricans, for example).

Diabetes autoantibody titers and C-peptide levels should not be tested at diagnosis. C-peptide concentrations have better discriminative value when there is a longer interval between the initial presentation and the test; these tests provide more accurate results when performed at a later point if the diagnosis remains unclear.[5]

Management. As is the case for children with type 1 diabetes, all children with type 2 diabetes should be referred to a specialist pediatric team and should receive ongoing and continuing multidisciplinary care within a specialist service.

Lifestyle changes are the mainstay of treatment for children and young people with type 2 diabetes. Weight management and eating habits should be discussed at every contact and the family should be offered dietetic support. If schemes are available locally, refer the individual, or preferably the whole family, for tailored exercise and lifestyle education.[5]

Weight and diet should always be explored with great sensitivity and social and cultural consideration. A sensitive approach is needed as these children and young people have an increased risk of psychological conditions that can affect their wellbeing.

Medication. NICE recommends standard-release metformin from diagnosis.[5] If this is poorly tolerated, a modified-release formulation can be trialed. The dose should be titrated slowly, and the child, young person or parent/carer advised that metformin should be taken at a mealtime. Liquid and powder formulations are available if a child is struggling to take the tablets, which are large.

The use of glucose-lowering therapies for children and young people is an area that is likely to develop as research evidence emerges. Given the high risk of erroneous diagnosis (i.e. type 1 diabetes or a rarer genetic cause of symptoms mistakenly diagnosed as type 2 diabetes), the initiation of glucose-lowering therapies should remain the responsibility of specialist pediatric diabetes teams. Guidance should always be sought where medication intolerance or glycemic control gives cause for concern.

Monitoring. Height and weight should be recorded at every clinic visit, with body mass index (BMI) plotted on a growth curve. Again, this should be carried out with sensitivity.

As for a child with type 1 diabetes, a glycosylated hemoglobin (HbA1c) target of 48 mmol/mol (6.5%) is ideal, though lifestyle, activities and comorbidities should be taken into account. Levels should be measured at 3-monthly intervals.

Complications. All children and young people diagnosed with type 2 diabetes should be screened for dyslipidemia and hypertension from diagnosis onward (Table 9.2). Children over the age of 12 years should also be referred for diabetic retinopathy and nephropathy screening. Ophthalmic referral should also be considered for children under 12 whose diabetes has been poorly controlled.

Pregnant women

The priorities for the care of women before conception and during pregnancy are outlined in Table 9.3. Better care is needed to improve pregnancy-related outcomes for this group. Women with diabetes experience a higher rate of miscarriage, stillbirth, premature birth, congenital anomalies and neonatal death.[6]

TABLE 9.2

Monitoring and treating hypertension and dyslipidemia in children and young people

Hypertension

- Measure blood pressure with an appropriately sized cuff
- Use 24-hour ambulatory blood pressure monitoring to confirm hypertension if resting measurements are repeatedly > 95th percentile for age and sex
- ACE inhibitors can be used for management*

Dyslipidemia

- Check and confirm with repeat test if necessary (fasting or non-fasting):
  - total cholesterol
  - HDL-cholesterol
  - non-HDL-cholesterol
  - triglyceride
- Statins can be used for management*

*Risk of pregnancy should be considered for sexually active young women.
ACE, angiotensin-converting enzyme; HDL, high-density lipoprotein.
Source: Thornton 2016.[4]

The 2018 National Pregnancy in Diabetes Audit revealed that, for the first time, more pregnant women with diabetes had type 2 diabetes than type 1.[6] Unfortunately, the audit also showed that, since 2014, there has been no improvement in the proportion of women achieving the recommended prepregnancy glycemic targets or taking the recommended higher dose of folic acid (5 mg): more than 60% of women with type 2 diabetes had a first trimester HbA1c above 48 mmol/mol and fewer than 25% took 5-mg folic acid.[6]

Babies of women with type 2 diabetes have an increased risk of congenital birth anomalies, macrosomia at birth and delayed growth during early pregnancy, which may reflect poor glucose control, a lower use of folic acid before conception and in early pregnancy or a higher likelihood of using (prescribed) teratogenic medications.[7,8]

TABLE 9.3

Priorities for the care of women with type 2 diabetes preconception and during pregnancy

Preconception

- Glucose is well managed, with HbA1c < 48 mmol/mol
- Safe and effective contraception is advised if HbA1c > 86 mmol/mol to avoid pregnancy until glucose control improves
- Folic acid at 5 mg/day is taken
- ACE inhibitors and ARBs should be stopped before conception or as soon as pregnancy is confirmed; an antihypertensive medication suitable for use in pregnancy should be substituted
- Statins should be stopped before conception or as soon as pregnancy is confirmed

During pregnancy

- Immediate contact with a joint diabetes and antenatal clinic should be offered, and contact with the joint clinic should continue every 1–2 weeks throughout pregnancy
- HbA1c should be measured at booking and in second and third trimesters (to assess the level of risk to the pregnancy)
- Good glycemic control is associated with reduced risk of adverse pregnancy outcomes; risk increases with rising HbA1c and particularly with HbA1c > 48 mmol/mol
- If no other complications, advise woman to have elective birth (induction or Cesarean section) between 37[+0] and 38[+6] weeks
- If complications for mother and/or fetus, consider elective birth before 37[+0] weeks

ACE, angiotensin-converting enzyme; ARB, angiotensin II receptor blocker; HbA1c, glycosylated hemoglobin.
Source. NICE 2015.[9]

Medication review, with discontinuation or substitution of teratogenic medications, should form a routine part of prepregnancy care for women actively planning pregnancy.

In particular, care needs to be taken to ensure that women at risk of adverse outcomes access services and support. In the 2018 National

Pregnancy in Diabetes Audit, more than half of women with type 2 diabetes were black, Asian or of mixed ethnicity. Women with type 2 diabetes also tended to be older and were more likely to be overweight and live in areas of social deprivation than women with type 1 diabetes.[6]

Retinal assessment. In both type 1 and type 2 diabetes, pregnancy may be associated with progression of diabetic retinopathy.[10,11] Imaging with mydriasis should be offered to women after their first antenatal clinic visit unless they have had an assessment within the previous 3 months. This should be repeated at 28 weeks, or at 16–20 weeks if diabetic retinopathy is present at booking.[9]

Practice point

Discuss risk of pregnancy when prescribing any drug for a woman of childbearing age.

Renal assessment, with measurement of serum creatinine and urinary albumin to creatinine ratio (ACR), should also be arranged at the first contact unless it has been performed in the last 3 months.[9] Estimated glomerular filtration rate (eGFR) should not be used in pregnancy.[9] Consider referring to a nephrologist if serum creatinine is at or above 120 μmol/L, urinary ACR is over 30 mg/mmol or total protein excretion exceeds 0.5 g/day.

Risk of pre-eclampsia. Women with type 2 diabetes have an increased risk of developing pre-eclampsia; the specialist multidisciplinary team caring for a woman may recommend her to take aspirin (acetylsalicylic acid), 75–150 mg daily, from 12 weeks until the birth.[12]

Monitoring fetal growth. Women should be offered ultrasound monitoring of fetal growth and amniotic fluid volume every 4 weeks from 28 to 36 weeks. Women with macrovascular disease and/or nephropathy should have an individualized monitoring plan.

Older people

The rising prevalence of type 2 diabetes and improving life expectancy mean that the number of older people living with diabetes is increasing globally. Age is an independent risk factor for type 2 diabetes, which is commonly diagnosed later in life, though many people diagnosed at a younger age are now living longer with diabetes.

Age and duration of diabetes are risk factors for all diabetes-related complications, but older people often face complications less commonly seen in younger people (Figure 9.1). Although many older people with diabetes live well, others suffer declining health, with multimorbidity, polypharmacy and social challenges impacting on wellbeing. Lifestyle intervention may be limited: musculoskeletal disorders may limit a person's ability to undertake physical activity and poor dentition or ill-fitting dentures may influence dietary choices. Holistic assessment that considers physical and mental health, and social and functional wellbeing is required to identify priorities, determine appropriate treatment goals and ensure person-

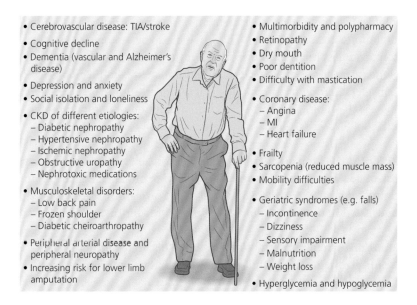

- Cerebrovascular disease: TIA/stroke
- Cognitive decline
- Dementia (vascular and Alzheimer's disease)
- Depression and anxiety
- Social isolation and loneliness
- CKD of different etiologies:
  – Diabetic nephropathy
  – Hypertensive nephropathy
  – Ischemic nephropathy
  – Obstructive uropathy
  – Nephrotoxic medications
- Musculoskeletal disorders:
  – Low back pain
  – Frozen shoulder
  – Diabetic cheiroarthropathy
- Peripheral arterial disease and peripheral neuropathy
- Increasing risk for lower limb amputation

- Multimorbidity and polypharmacy
- Retinopathy
- Dry mouth
- Poor dentition
- Difficulty with mastication
- Coronary disease:
  – Angina
  – MI
  – Heart failure
- Frailty
- Sarcopenia (reduced muscle mass)
- Mobility difficulties
- Geriatric syndromes (e.g. falls)
  – Incontinence
  – Dizziness
  – Sensory impairment
  – Malnutrition
  – Weight loss
- Hyperglycemia and hypoglycemia

Figure 9.1 Diabetes in later life may be associated with a wide range of comorbidities and complications, many of which are interlinked and will impact on each other.[13] CKD, chronic kidney disease; MI, myocardial infarction; TIA, transient ischemic attack.

centered care. Older people are also more vulnerable to treatment side effects and, in particular, hypoglycemia, which needs to be considered when prescribing glucose-lowering therapies.[13]

For some older people, particularly when type 2 diabetes is diagnosed relatively later in life, the classic macrovascular and microvascular complications of type 2 diabetes may have less impact than in younger people, with frailty and muscle loss being potentially more important.[14] Overaggressive management of blood glucose may adversely affect functional ability, with negative consequences for the person's quality of life. For example, a US observational study of older people with diabetes living in the community (mean age 80 years) found that those with an HbA1c of 8.0–8.9% (64–74 mmol/mol) had better functional outcomes at 2 years than those with an HbA1c in the range 7.0–7.9% (53–63 mmol/mol).[15]

Diagnosis may be incidental – up to half of older people with type 2 diabetes may be asymptomatic – and an older person should be checked for signs of diabetes at every opportunity (e.g. admission to hospital or a nursing home). Signs vary widely. A person may have an unexpected fall or develop memory problems, general tiredness or non-specific illness that may be ascribed to old age. Up to 1 in 3 older residents in care homes are affected by diabetes.[16]

Management approaches should consider the increasing complexity of type 2 diabetes in older people, the likely changing health status of the individual as they age and the impact of polypharmacy and comorbidities. In particular, cognitive impairment, dementia or frailty have a bearing on management. There is growing concern that intensive glucose-lowering strategies, particularly where medications associated with a higher risk of hypoglycemia are used, may not be beneficial for frail older people. Liaison with specialists in diabetes care for older adults can help to optimize individual management plans to overcome issues with communication, overprescribing and unnecessary hospital admissions. Suggestions to de-escalate or discontinue medications should be made sensitively to the individual and their family and the reasoning should be made clear. Care should be taken that the proposed action is not seen as a decision not to treat. Some of the issues related to medication to be considered when managing elderly patients with type 2 diabetes are summarized in Table 9.4.

TABLE 9.4

Potential risks with glucose-lowering medications that may adversely affect older people

- Thiazolidinediones: increased risk of heart failure, edema, bone fractures and weight gain
- DPP-4 inhibitors: saxagliptin has been associated with heart failure; all others, except linagliptin, require dose adjustment with declining eGFR
- SGLT2 inhibitors: promote an osmotic diuresis with glucosuria, so there is a risk of genitourinary infections, volume depletion, dehydration, orthostatic hypotension and AKI. Note that some have upper age limits for the licensed indication. Cautions for DKA and lower limb amputations are as previously described (see Table 5.3)
- GLP-1RAs: may cause weight loss, increasing frailty, and exacerbate sarcopenia
- Sulfonylurea and insulin therapies: risk of hypoglycemia with potentially serious consequences

AKI, acute kidney injury; DKA, diabetic ketoacidosis; DPP-4, dipeptidyl peptidase-4; eGFR, estimated glomerular filtration rate; GLP-1RA, glucagon-like peptide-1 receptor agonist; SGLT2, sodium–glucose cotransporter 2.
Source: Hambling et al. 2019.[13]

Cognitive impairment and dementia, including both vascular dementia and Alzheimer's disease, are more common in older people with diabetes, with onset at a slightly younger age than is seen in people without diabetes. There is no evidence that intensive glycemic management reduces the risk of cognitive impairment or dementia; conversely, the presence of cognitive impairment or dementia increases the risk of hypoglycemia, which in turn risks exacerbating cognitive function. Overintensive glycemic management should be avoided in people with cognitive impairment, particularly with medications such as sulfonylureas or insulin therapies, which carry a higher risk of hypoglycemia.[13]

Frailty can be assessed using a number of tools and scoring systems: the Electronic Frailty Index (eFI) is now widely available on clinical systems in primary care and can be used to identify vulnerable people. A clinical assessment, such as the 4-meter gait speed or a timed

TABLE 9.5

The FRAIL scale

Assessment	Question
Fatigue	Is the person fatigued?
Resistance	Can he or she walk up one flight of stairs?
Aerobic	Can he or she walk for about 3 minutes?
Illnesses	Does he or she have > 5 illnesses?
Loss of weight	Has he or she lost > 5% of their bodyweight in the last 6 months?

Number of positive answers	Outcome
1–2	Pre-frailty
≥ 3	Frail

Source: Abellan Van Kan et al. 2008.[17]

get-up-and-go test, should be included when frailty is assessed, though such tests may not always be practical. Alternatives to the eFI include the FRAIL scale (Table 9.5) and the Clinical Frailty Scale, which also assesses cognitive frailty.

Hypoglycemia may present differently in older people: blunted physiological responses may mean that typical adrenergic responses (sweating, palpitations, increased heart rate) are not manifest, so blood glucose levels fall further and neuroglycopenic symptoms appear (confusion, sleepiness, agitation). These symptoms may be misinterpreted, particularly in those with cognitive impairment, further delaying treatment.

Where possible, glucose-lowering therapies associated with a higher risk of hypoglycemia, such as sulfonylureas and insulin therapies, should be avoided. Where these medications carrying a higher risk of hypoglycemia are considered necessary, it is important that carers and family are informed of the risks, understand what symptoms to be alert to, have access to capillary glucose testing and know what actions to take. Any episode of hypoglycemia should prompt a subsequent clinical review. The consequences of hypoglycemia in an older person can be serious – increasing the risk for cardiovascular events, falls, fractures and head injury – and potentially fatal.[13]

Fit 'biologically young' older adults can be treated as younger adults. A treatment target of 58 mmol/mol (7.5%) or below is reasonable. If glycemic control is good, the medical regimen can continue unless there is evidence of overtreatment.[14] In general, avoid starting a new agent that may cause hypoglycemia or weight loss.

Moderate to severely frail older adults. A treatment target of 64 mmol/mol (8.0%) or below is appropriate. If HbA1c is below 58 mmol/mol (7.5%) with glucose-lowering therapies, sulfonylureas can be reduced or discontinued; thiazolidinediones should be avoided where there is risk of heart failure, and metformin used with caution and dose adjustment in those with renal impairment. Dipeptidyl peptidase-4 (DPP-4) inhibitors are generally well tolerated, though dose adjustment may be required in individuals with renal impairment, and saxagliptin should be avoided in those at risk of heart failure. Sodium–glucose cotransporter 2 (SGLT2) inhibitors can be helpful in the presence of heart failure, but caution is required to avoid volume depletion, particularly when diuretics are also prescribed. Practitioners should also be aware that use of SGLT2 inhibitors is associated with an increased risk of genital mycotic infections.[18]

For those using insulin, a review that includes hypoglycemia risk assessment should be undertaken and, where possible, the insulin regimen simplified. Longer-acting insulins with relatively lower hypoglycemia risk may be more suitable.[13,14]

Very severely frail older adults. A treatment target below 70 mmol/mol (8.5%) is appropriate. The above guidance regarding glucose-lowering therapies also applies here, though a de-escalation threshold of 64 mmol/mol (8.0%) has been proposed, at or below which the reduction or withdrawal of sulfonylureas and short-acting insulins should be considered because of the risks associated with hypoglycemia. Similarly, the timings of administration of neutral protamine Hagedorn (NPH) insulin and its continuing suitability should also be assessed for those at this threshold. Where necessary, once-daily morning NPH insulin or an insulin associated with a lower incidence of hypoglycemia, such as a second-generation basal insulin analog, may be preferred.[19,20]

Individuals with hepatic impairment

Non-alcoholic fatty liver disease (NAFLD) has a strong association with insulin resistance, obesity and type 2 diabetes. As many as 70% of people with type 2 diabetes may be affected, and there is evidence that liver disease may progress more rapidly in people with type 2 diabetes.[21,22] It is important to note that NAFLD affects children as well as adults and is reported as evident at diagnosis in 37% of children with type 2 diabetes.[1]

Although NAFLD is, in itself, relatively benign, its importance lies in the risk that it will progress to more serious liver disease. A significant 30% of those with NAFLD will progress to non-alcoholic steatohepatitis, with liver inflammation; of these, approximately one-third will develop cirrhosis, with increased morbidity and mortality.[22] In addition to the risk of progressive liver disease, NAFLD is associated with increased risk for cardiovascular disease.[22]

Diagnosis of NAFLD is difficult as there is no single test. Liver biopsy remains the gold standard, but this is impractical for most individuals. Liver function tests (LFTs) are neither sensitive nor specific and normal LFTs, even in the presence of significant liver disease, are common. Although normal values do not exclude a diagnosis, 70% of people with NAFLD and type 2 diabetes have values outside the normal range.[22]

Ultrasound has acceptable specificity and sensitivity for moderate to severe fatty liver; it can be considered, though there is no universally accepted definition of steatosis based on ultrasound findings. New imaging techniques aimed at better assessing liver disease are being developed, though at present these are inconsistently available and, as yet, no single imaging method has emerged as the preferred test.[23]

Liver fibrosis can be assessed using biomarkers. The Fibrosis-4 (FIB-4) calculation can be performed in primary care.[24] Although not universally available, NICE recommends the enhanced liver fibrosis (ELF) test to identify individuals with high-risk fibrosis.[25] ELF combines the assessment of tissue inhibitor of metalloproteinase 1 (TIMP-1), amino-terminal propeptide of type III procollagen (PIIINP) and hyaluronic acid in a single score. A diagnosis of NAFLD and an ELF score equal to or above 10.51 indicates advanced liver fibrosis.[25]

Management of NAFLD depends on the degree of liver disease.

Low ELF score. Lifestyle modification is recommended for those with low risk of progression to advanced liver disease (ELF score < 10.51), as individuals with NAFLD have a heightened risk of cardiovascular disease. A low-energy diet (600–800 kcal reduction in intake) may be beneficial as there is evidence that weight loss of 5–10% can reduce inflammation of the liver as well as improve insulin sensitivity. Exercise can also benefit liver health. Patients should be counseled to avoid misusing alcohol.

Blood pressure and blood lipids should be monitored, and hypertension and dyslipidemia should be treated (see chapter 6). Statins can be used safely in this patient group unless alanine aminotransferase (ALT) is at or over three times the upper limit of normal.[22]

High ELF score. NICE recommends that people with a high ELF score (≥ 10.51) should be referred to specialist services.[25] Thiazolidinediones and vitamin E have been suggested as treatments to slow the progression of liver disease in individuals with advanced fibrosis, but these are best considered within secondary care.

Considerations for glucose-lowering therapies. Given the importance of the liver in the metabolism of medications, it is advisable to manage a patient with type 2 diabetes and NAFLD within a multidisciplinary team.

Key points – special populations

- More children are being diagnosed with type 2 diabetes. A child with type 2 diabetes may be asymptomatic or identified via testing in the community; recurrent genital/perineal infections should prompt diabetes testing.
- Risk factors for type 2 diabetes in a child or young person include family history, obesity, black or Asian ethnic background, lack of insulin requirement and evidence of insulin resistance.

Key points – special populations (CONTINUED)

- Care of a child or young person with type 2 diabetes should be delivered with sensitivity and support as these individuals have a heightened risk of psychological illness.
- All children with diabetes should be looked after within specialist pediatric diabetes services.
- All women with diabetes and of childbearing age should be counseled about the need for good glucose control and higher-dose (5 mg) folic acid before conception and to use effective contraception until glucose is well managed (even when not actively planning pregnancy).
- The risk to the pregnancy increases with glycosylated hemoglobin (HbA1c) above 48 mmol/mol.
- Teratogenic drugs (angiotensin-converting enzyme [ACE] inhibitors, angiotensin II receptor blockers [ARBs] and statins) should be proactively stopped/replaced when pregnancy is planned or as soon as pregnancy is confirmed.
- When managing an older person with type 2 diabetes, holistic assessment that considers physical and mental health and social and functional wellbeing should be adopted to determine priorities and to ensure person-centered care.
- Glycemic goals should be agreed and intensive glycemic management avoided; an aggressive approach to blood glucose control may not be optimal for quality of life.
- Glucose-lowering options for older people should be tailored to overall wellbeing; frailty and cognitive function should be assessed, with consideration given to comorbidities, the effect of polypharmacy and the side effects of medications, including the risk of hypoglycemia.
- Non-alcoholic fatty liver disease is common in people with type 2 diabetes, but it can be challenging to diagnose; the enhanced liver fibrosis biomarker score can be used to assess hepatic fibrosis.
- Lifestyle modification, with exercise and weight loss, can benefit the risk of progression of non-alcoholic fatty liver disease and improve insulin sensitivity.

References

1. Candler TP, Mahmoud O, Lynn RM et al. Continuing rise of type 2 diabetes incidence in children and young people in the UK. *Diabet Med* 2018;35:737–44.

2. Hannon TS, Arslanian SA. The changing face of diabetes in youth: lessons learned from studies of type 2 diabetes. *Ann N Y Acad Sci* 2015;1353:113–37.

3. Dart AB, Martens PJ, Rigatto C et al. Earlier onset of complications in youth with type 2 diabetes. *Diabetes Care* 2014;37:436–43.

4. Thornton H. New NICE guidance: changes in practice for multidisciplinary teams. Part 2: type 2 diabetes in children and young people. *J Diabetes Nurs* 2016;20: 210–12.

5. National Institute for Health and Care Excellence. Diabetes (type 1 and type 2) in children and young people: diagnosis and management: NG18. London: NICE, 2015.

6. NHS Diabetes Audit. National Pregnancy in Diabetes Audit Report 2018. *NHS Digital*, 2019. https:// digital.nhs.uk/data-and-information/ publications/statistical/national- pregnancy-in-diabetes-audit/ national-pregnancy-in-diabetes- annual-report-2018, last accessed 8 July 2020.

7. Geurtsen ML, van Soest EEL, Voerman E et al. High maternal early-pregnancy blood glucose levels are associated with altered fetal growth and increased risk of adverse birth outcomes. *Diabetologia* 2019;62:1880–90.

8. Murphy HR, Bell R, Cartwright C et al. Improved pregnancy outcomes in women with type 1 and type 2 diabetes but substantial clinic-to- clinic variations: a prospective nationwide study. *Diabetologia* 2017;60:1668–77.

9. National Institute for Health and Care Excellence. Diabetes in pregnancy: management from preconception to the postnatal period: NG3. London. NICE, 2015.

10. Vestgaard M, Ringholm L, Laugesen CS et al. Pregnancy-induced sight-threatening diabetic retinopathy in women with type 1 diabetes. *Diabet Med* 2010;27:431–5.

11. Rasmussen KL, Laugesen CS, Ringholm L et al. Progression of diabetic retinopathy during pregnancy in women with type 2 diabetes. *Diabetologia* 2010;53: 1076–83.

12. National Institute for Health and Care Excellence. Hypertension in pregnancy: diagnosis and management: NG133. London: NICE, 2019.

13. Hambling CE, Khunti K, Cos X et al. Factors influencing safe glucose-lowering in older adults with type 2 diabetes: a person-centred approach to individualised (PROACTIVE) glycemic goals for older people: a position statement of Primary Care Diabetes Europe. *Prim Care Diabetes* 2019;13:330–52.

14. Strain WD, Hope SV, Green A et al. Type 2 diabetes mellitus in older people: a brief statement of key principles of modern day management including the assessment of frailty. A national collaborative stakeholder initiative. *Diabet Med* 2018;35:838–45.

15. Yau CK, Eng C, Cenzer IS et al. Glycosylated hemoglobin and functional decline in community-dwelling nursing home-eligible elderly adults with diabetes mellitus. *J Am Geriatr Soc* 2012;60:1215–21.

16. Sinclair AJ, Gadsby R, Abdelhafiz AH et al. Failing to meet the needs of generations of care home residents with diabetes: a review of the literature and a call for action. *Diabet Med* 2018;35:1144–56.

17. Abellan Van Kan G, Rolland Y, Bergman H et al. The I.A.N.A. task force on frailty assessment of older people in clinical practice. *J Nutr Heal Aging* 2008;12:29–37.

18. Lega IC, Bronskill SE, Campitelli MA et al. Sodium glucose cotransporter 2 inhibitors and risk of genital mycotic and urinary tract infection: a population-based study of older women and men with diabetes. *Diabetes Obes Metab* 2019;21:2394–404.

19. Wysham C, Bhargava A, Chaykin L et al. Effect of insulin degludec vs insulin glargine U100 on hypoglycemia in patients with type 2 diabetes: the SWITCH 2 randomized clinical trial. *JAMA* 2017;318:45–56.

20. Ritzel R, Harris SB, Baron H et al. A randomized controlled trial comparing efficacy and safety of insulin glargine 300 units/mL versus 100 units/mL in older people with type 2 diabetes: results from the SENIOR study. *Diabetes Care* 2018;41:dc180168.

21. Vernon G, Baranova A, Younossi ZM. Systematic review: the epidemiology and natural history of non-alcoholic fatty liver disease and non-alcoholic steatohepatitis in adults. *Aliment Pharmacol Ther* 2011;34:274–85.

22. Wainwright P. Non-alcoholic fatty liver disease and diabetes: diagnosis, assessment and management. *Clin Pharm* 2017;9. doi: 10.1211/CP.2017.20202993.

23. Graffy PM, Pickhardt PJ. Quantification of hepatic and visceral fat by CT and MR imaging: relevance to the obesity epidemic, metabolic syndrome and NAFLD. *Br J Radiol* 2016;89:20151024.

24. Adler M, Gulbis B, Moreno C et al. The predictive value of FIB-4 versus FibroTest, APRI, FibroIndex and Forns index to noninvasively estimate fibrosis in hepatitis C and nonhepatitis C liver diseases. *Hepatology* 2008;47:762–3.

25. National Institute for Health and Care Excellence. Non-alcoholic fatty liver disease (NAFLD): assessment and management: NG49. London: NICE, 2016.

Useful resources

Organizations

Diabetes UK
www.diabetes.org.uk

International Diabetes Federation
www.idf.org

European Association for the Study
of Diabetes
www.easd.org

American Diabetes Association
www.diabetes.org

Management guidelines

National Institute for Health and Care
Excellence, Type 2 diabetes in adults:
management; NG28 (2015)
www.nice.org.uk/guidance/NG28

Scottish Intercollegiate Guidelines
Network, Management of diabetes;
SIGN 154 (2017) and 116 (2010)
www.sign.ac.uk/sign-116-and-154-
diabetes.html; quick reference guide
www.sign.ac.uk/assets/Qrg116.pdf

American Diabetes Association/
European Association for the Study
of Diabetes

Davies M, D'Alessio D, Fradkin J et al.
Management of hyperglycemia in type 2
diabetes, 2018. A consensus report by
the American Diabetes Association
(ADA) and the European Association for
the Study of Diabetes (EASD). *Diabetes
Care* 2018;41:2669–701.

Buse JB, Wexler DJ, Tsapas A et al.
2019 update to: Management of
hyperglycaemia in type 2 diabetes,
2018. A consensus report by the
American Diabetes Association (ADA)
and the European Association for the
Study of Diabetes (EASD). *Diabetologia*
2020;63:221–8.

American Diabetes Association.
Standards of Medical Care in Diabetes
(2020)
https://care.diabetesjournals.org/
content/43/Supplement_1 (an
abridged version for primary care
providers is available at https://
clinical.diabetesjournals.org/content/
diaclin/38/1/10.full.pdf)

NICE Quality Standards relevant to type 2 diabetes

QS5 Chronic kidney disease in adults
(2011, updated 2017)
www.nice.org.uk/guidance/qs5

QS6 Diabetes in adults (2011,
updated 2016)
www.nice.org.uk/guidance/qs6

QS9 Chronic heart failure in adults
(2011, updated 2018)
www.nice.org.uk/guidance/qs9

QS52 Peripheral arterial disease (2014)
www.nice.org.uk/guidance/qs52

QS100 Cardiovascular risk assessment
and lipid modification (2015)
www.nice.org.uk/guidance/qs100

QS111 Obesity in adults: prevention
and lifestyle weight management
programmes (2016)
www.nice.org.uk/guidance/qs111

Index